Pilates'
Body Conditioning

A Program Based on the Techniques of

Joseph Pilates

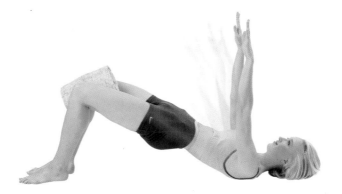

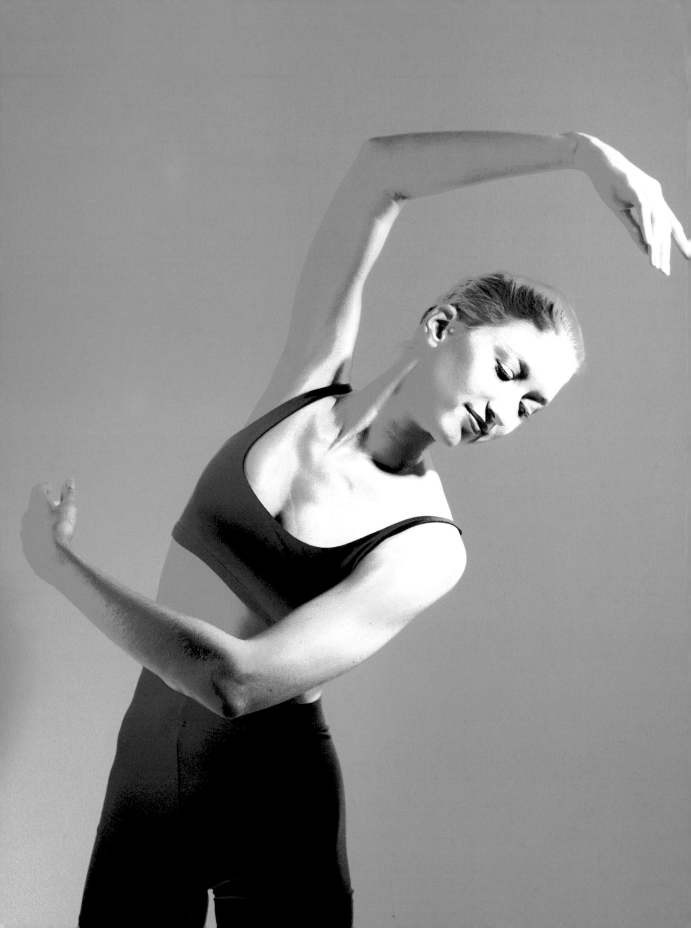

Pilates'
Body Conditioning

A Program Based on the Techniques of
Joseph Pilates

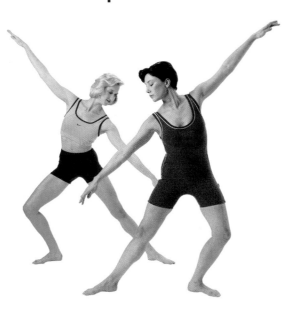

Anna Selby & Alan Herdman

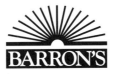

BARRON'S

All inquiries should be addressed to:
Barron's Educational Series, Inc.
250 Wireless Boulevard
Hauppauge, NY 11788
http://www.barronseduc.com

International Standard Book No: 0-7641-1627-4

Library of Congress Catalog Card No. 00-101227

Printed in Singapore

9 8 7 6 5 4 3 2 1

Important Note

The techniques, ideas, and suggestions in this book are to be used at the reader's
sole discretion and risk. Always observe the cautions given, and consult a doctor if
in doubt about a medical condition.

How to use this book

This book has been designed as a progressive course. Your program starts with a self-assessment to help you identify your strengths and weaknesses, and locate important and often forgotten muscles. It is a good idea to go back to these self-assessment exercises over the weeks to see how you have changed – always an uplifting experience!

The warm-up that starts on page 48 is common to all levels – do it at the start of every session to help you focus and become body-aware before you go on to the more complex movements that follow. Each level works every part of your body but you will, of course, find that some parts of you are stronger or more flexible than others. However, it is best to be able to do all of the exercises in each level comfortably before going on to the next. Within each level, some exercises are harder than others, so leave ones such as the advanced abdominals in level three until you are really strong. It is particularly important to build up the "girdle of strength," the pelvic and abdominal support for the whole body, gradually so that you can take on more difficult movements safely. If your abdominal muscles bulge or quiver, stop! This is a warning that they aren't strong enough yet to perform the exercise. In this case, do fewer repetitions or try not to go so far.

The number of repetitions is specified in each exercise. Don't be tempted to do more – it is quality and precision that count in Joseph Pilates' technique, not quantity. Ideally, aim for three sessions a week, with a rest day between each one.

The exercises in this book are all nonaerobic and, to supplement them, we recommend regular aerobic exercise. Brisk walking is easy to incorporate into your daily routine, and swimming and cycling are also ideal. Running or jogging, however, are all too likely to cause injury, notably to knees and backs, particularly if you run on a hard surface, such as a pavement. Try to take two or three 20-minute exercise periods each week, choosing exercise that leaves you slightly out of breath.

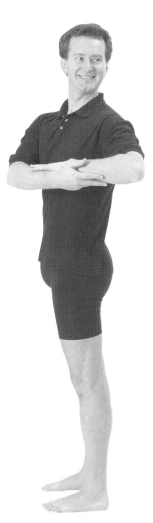

Contents

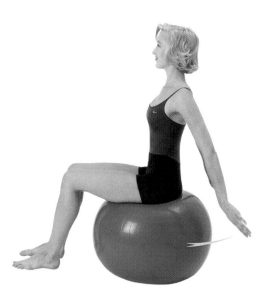

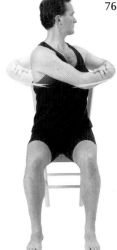

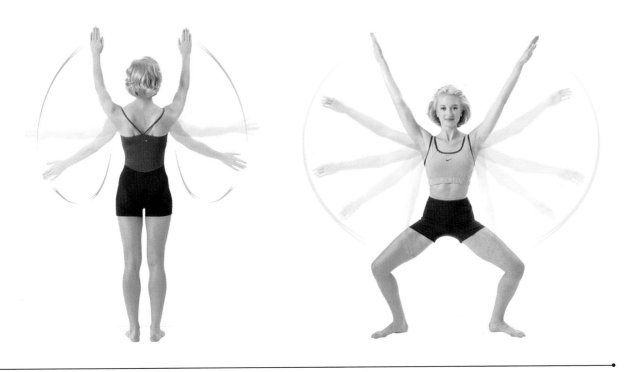

Foreword

I have been practicing Joseph Pilates' exercising technique at Alan's studio for about seventeen years. I have also been "floored" and "at it" in hotel rooms all over the world. His exercises are precisely the kind of exercises I need and like. You don't have to dance around; you merely tone all the muscles in the body. So many of the wonderful new exercise routines introduced these days are found to be harmful from various points of view a year or two later.

Apart from a general feeling of well-being created by doing Pilates' exercises, I find them invaluable in keeping me out of the osteopath's hands. I have a back problem exacerbated by the practice of judo on the cement studio floor during "The Avengers" and provided the muscles in my back are kept strong and flexible, I find my vertebrae remain exactly where they should be.

I wrote a book a couple of years ago about how to stay vigorous, stylish, and groomed, and one of the most vital chapters involved Joseph Pilates' exercises. Indeed, it includes a jolly picture of Alan and me, as he was good enough to help me with all the appropriate names for the muscles. I remember saying in the book that all that one needed to exercise efficiently at home was a kitchen chair, a cushion, a book, a couple of cans of soup, and a small towel. That's what's so wonderful about these exercises — you need no expensive equipment and you can do it anywhere – well almost anywhere.

Alan is a wonderful instructor, and quite strict. There is no point in vaguely waltzing through exercises; you must concentrate and be sure that you achieve the object of the exercise. A shorter period of time with the job done thoroughly is worth more than twice the time rushed and inefficiently performed.

Before I start my exercises I often think, "Oh, no!" but at the end I'm upright, walking tall, and feeling marvelous and vibrant (a favorite word of my old stablemate, Patrick Macnee).

I can leave you in Alan's hands with total confidence. Go to it and it is one decision you will have made in life, and kept to, that you will never regret.

Honor Blackman

About the authors

Anna Selby has been involved in many forms of dance and exercise, including ballet, Martha Graham technique, yoga, and Tai Chi. However, her first interest was Joseph Pilates' technique, and in 1985 her *Woman's Workout Book* was the first book in the UK to include the subject. She has subsequently written nine more books, mostly on exercise and health, including aromatherapy and Chinese herbal medicine. Having been a features reporter for BBC radio's immensely popular "Woman's Hour," she is now a freelance feature writer for a variety of UK newspapers and magazines, including *The Times*, the *Daily Telegraph*, the *Evening Standard*, and *Harpers and Queen*.

Alan Herdman is the leading practitioner of Joseph Pilates' technique in the UK. Having learned the method in New York, he introduced Joseph Pilates' technique to London in the early 1970s, and set up the first studio dedicated to it in England. His previous training was with London Contemporary Dance in the Martha Graham technique, and he was also trained as a teacher in Laban Dance Drama. In addition to his London studio, he has established several others around the world, including Sweden and Israel. As a teacher trainer, he has passed on his knowledge and expertise to many teachers of Joseph Pilates' technique, as well as to dancers of the London School of Contemporary Dance, the English National Ballet, the Houston Ballet, and Israel's Bat-Dor Dance Company. He also works with the English National Ballet School and Company, the Royal Academy of Dance, Elmhurst Ballet School, and is a guest teacher every year in Japan and the United States.

Introduction

Joseph Pilates was fond of pointing out that he had invented a technique that was fifty years ahead of its time.

Given its enormous popularity now, we can only concur. It has spread from a single studio in New York frequented by professional dancers to a technique with worldwide appeal practiced by people from every age group and background.

The reasons for such success are rooted in the fact that, quite simply, it works. After the endless exercise fads of recent decades, this technique has emerged as the one most likely to give you the body you want in the safest possible way.

Most forms of sport and exercise concentrate on the larger stronger muscles and, as these get stronger and bulkier, the smaller weaker muscles are forgotten. In Joseph Pilates' technique, however, these weaker muscles – often ones that many people are not even aware of – are strengthened, while the larger muscles become increasingly toned and sleek, creating a balanced, lithe, integrated body. Locating these smaller muscles and learning how to use them requires a great deal of concentration, control, and precision – and, for this reason, Joseph Pilates' technique is commonly referred to as "thinking exercise." It requires an unusual synchronization of mind and body and this, in turn, results in a sense of wholeness and integration more commonly associated with eastern meditative and movement techniques.

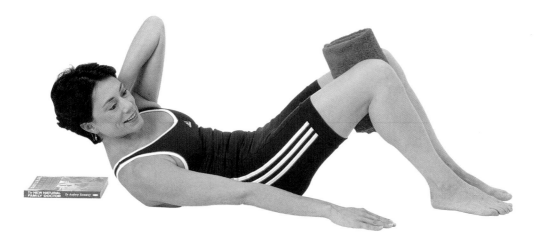

Concentration is one of the six basic principles of Joseph Pilates' technique, reflected in his own favorite quotation from the poet Schiller, "It is the mind itself that builds the body." The other basic principles are breathing, control, centering, flowing movement, and precision. Because the exercises are so controlled, they are very safe; the technique is ideal, for instance, for those in rehabilitation after an accident. It is also perfect for any age, as is made evident by the numerous seventy-year-olds in Alan Herdman's London studio!

This is the technique in which you finally get to know your own body. As you learn through the exercises how to use it properly, your posture improves, your muscles become more toned, your joints more mobile, and your body shape becomes more balanced, poised, and elongated. This is achieved not by endless repetitions of mind-numbingly boring exercises, but by minimal movements that use controlled muscles rather than momentum. At first it may seem that little is happening, especially if you are used to aerobic classes or gyms where you lift heavy weights. However, to be able to use your body correctly, you have to become aware of it as an integrated entity; many of the early exercises in this book are about locating forgotten muscles and learning how to move your body to achieve the best possible results.

By working your way through the levels in this book, you can expect to develop the body you have always wanted. You may not necessarily lose weight – muscles weigh more than fat – but you will flatten your stomach, tone and elongate your limbs, lift your buttocks, and have the poise and elegance of a dancer. Best of all, the lessons learned here spill over into everyday life, so even the most routine activities – sitting, walking, or standing – become infused with grace and balance.

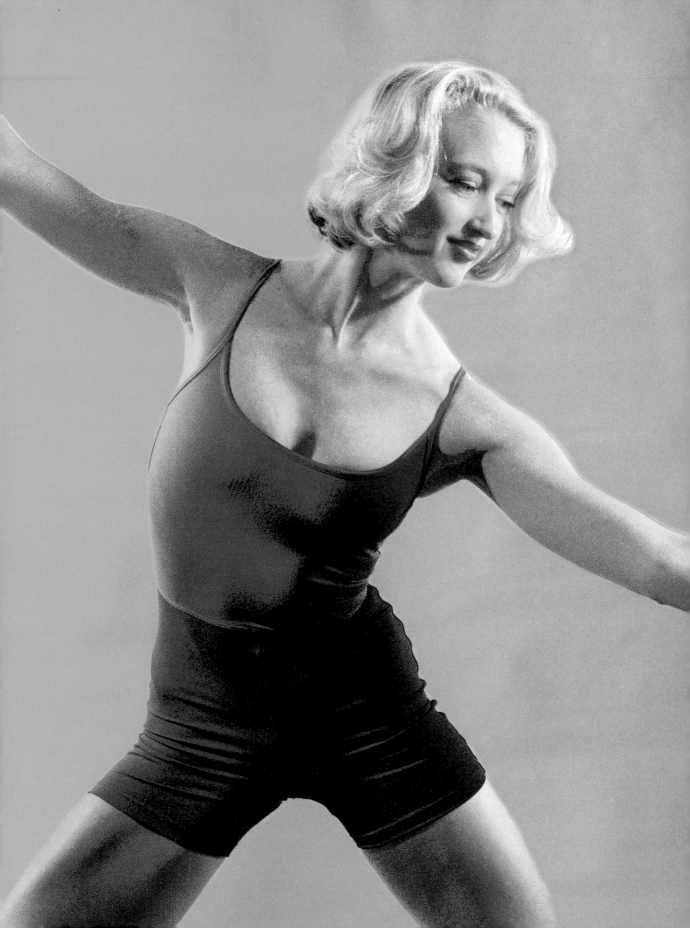

Chapter One

The Birth of Pilates' Technique

Joseph Hubertus Pilates was born in 1880 near Düsseldorf in Germany. He was a frail child, regarded as prone to tuberculosis.

However, so determined was he to improve his physical condition, instead of being limited by it, that he worked relentlessly at bodybuilding and conditioning until, by the age of fourteen, he was posing as a model for anatomical drawings. He went on to become an avid sportsman in various fields: He was a gymnast, a skier, a diver, a boxer, even a circus performer. In 1912 he left his native Germany for England where he became a professional boxer and taught self-defense to detectives at Scotland Yard.

When World War I broke out two years later, the British authorities interned him as a German national. He decided to use his enforced leisure to develop his ideas about health and physical fitness. His influences were wide-ranging, to say the least, embracing everything from yoga to the study of animal movements. He instructed his fellow internees in his evolving techniques, claiming that because of this not one of them died in the influenza epidemic of 1918!

After the war, he returned to Germany, and worked with most of the pioneers of movement technique but closest with Rudolf von Laban, the creator of the form of dance notation most widely used today. At the same time, Joseph Pilates was working as a trainer for the Hamburg police force. This time,

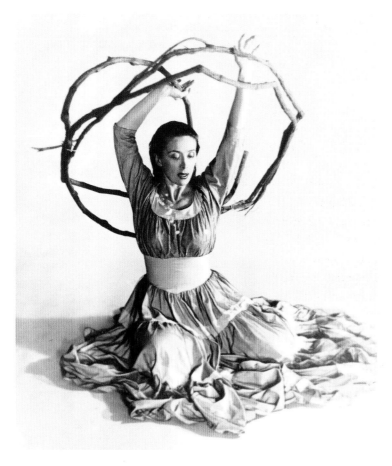

MARTHA GRAHAM
American choreographer, dancer, teacher, and pioneer of modern dance, as she appears in *Salem Shore* (c.1924).

however, he did not stay in Germany long. In 1923 he left for New York to set up his first studio with his wife Clara.

Pilates' method was an immediate success in America, particularly among dancers – Martha Graham and George Balanchine were early converts. Dancers, necessarily prone to injury, soon discovered, too, that rehabilitation using Pilates' exercises led to a swifter recovery, and this at a time when the therapeutic effects of immediate rehabilitation had not been recognized. However, during his internment, Pilates had worked for a while as a nurse. In this capacity, he had experimented with springs attached to hospital beds so that patients could begin to work on toning their muscles even before they could get up.

Again using springs as resistance, Pilates designed the machine he called his "Universal Reformer," a sliding, horizontal bed that can be used with up to four springs, according to the exercise and the strength of the individual. Today, the descendant of the Universal Reformer is usually known as a plié machine and it is still central to the body conditioning studio. Other machines were developed, and the method grew and spread over the years.

Alan Herdman introduced the method to Britain in the early 1970s, after studying Joseph Pilates' technique in New York with two of his foremost disciples, Bob Fitzgerald and Carola Trier, who were personally trained by Joseph Pilates. Alan's studio in London is now an internationally respected center for the technique. Over the years since Joseph Pilates set up his studio, his technique has been developed in a variety of ways. Some teachers have used a percussive, fast-paced method with effort coinciding with inhaling. This tends to build bulky muscles at the expense of the less-developed ones. One of the most distinctive features of Alan Herdman's teaching is the focused breathing, where all effort is placed on exhaling, leading both to a supremely balanced and poised body, and a relaxed, focused mind. All movements are extremely slow and rhythmic, allowing weaker muscles to be located and well worked.

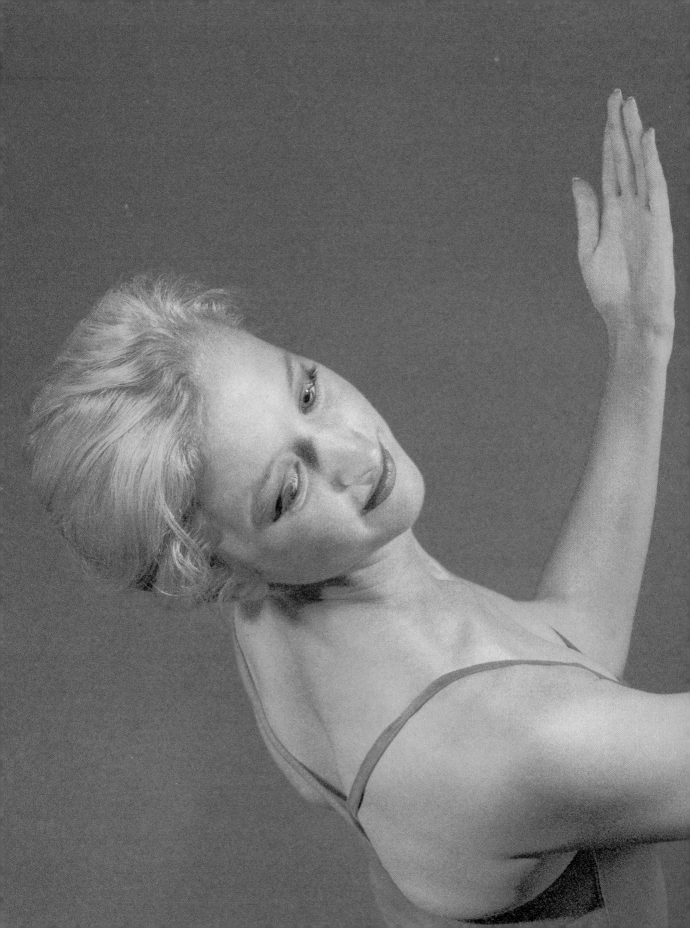

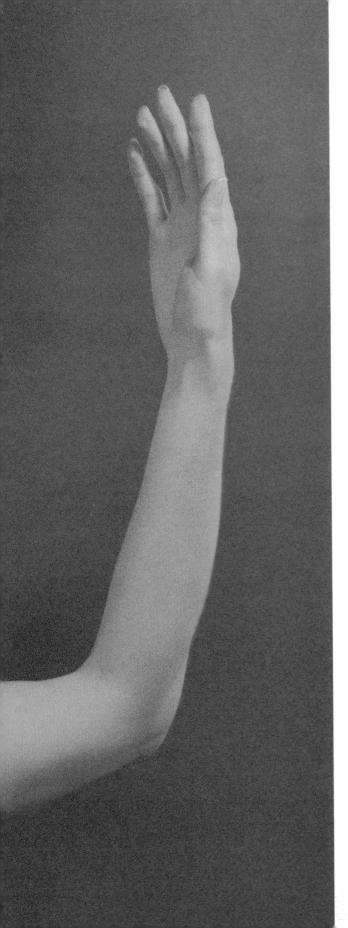

Chapter Two

Your Body Basics

Before you begin to exercise, take time to assess your own body. We all have bad habits of posture or in the ways we move and it is vital to recognize and correct these before you begin.

One of the most important aspects of Joseph Pilates' technique is that it starts with fundamentals – posture and breathing – and all the exercises build on these foundations. Body Basics shows you how to assess your own posture and breathing with simple exercises that use either the floor or a mirror. Take time on these basic assessments before you begin to exercise – it will repay you tenfold when you get started!

Muscle groups of the body

In Joseph Pilates' technique, you use your muscles in a very precise and focused way. The emphasis is on the quality of the movement, often with many muscles being used in synchronization within any given exercise. Some of these are likely to be weak from lack of use, so much so that they may be difficult to locate. These pages show where the main muscle groups are. For a further explanation of how to use them in Joseph Pilates' technique, see the glossary on p. 139.

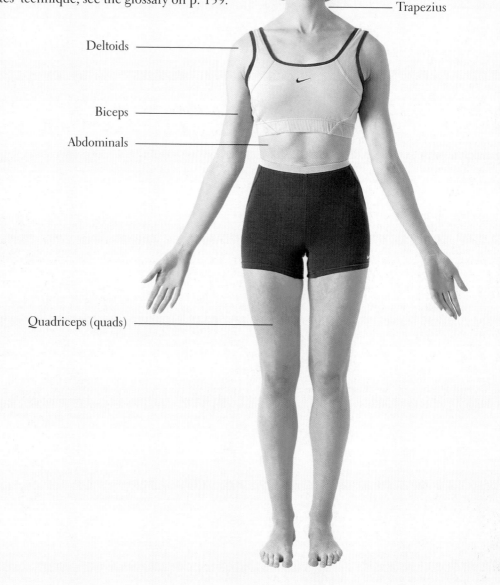

Trapezius

Deltoids

Biceps

Abdominals

Quadriceps (quads)

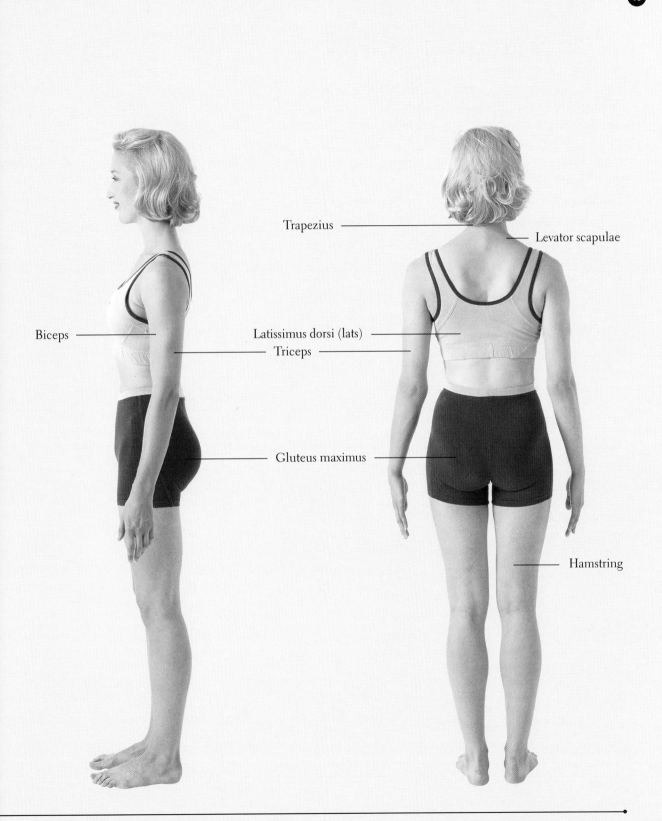

Trapezius

Levator scapulae

Biceps

Latissimus dorsi (lats)

Triceps

Gluteus maximus

Hamstring

Good and bad posture

One of the great benefits of Joseph Pilates' technique is the elongated posture you achieve, with the loose, graceful shape of a dancer. Beyond appearances, however, good posture is vital while you're exercising, and it helps you get the maximum benefit from your workout. If you don't hold on to your abdominal muscles while you exercise, you're in danger of straining your back, while moving your arms from tense neck and shoulders will only increase tension, and will probably give you a headache as well!

The photograph of bad posture on this page may look somewhat exaggerated, and you would be very unfortunate to start off with all of the problems shown, but it does indicate the most common postural faults, and it is a good idea to start your own assessment in front of a mirror, comparing your own body shape with the one shown here. Look both front and sideways into the mirror and go through this checklist, at your own pace.

Head and neck

Does your chin jut out or tilt upward? If so, it is pulling your spine out of alignment and shortening the muscles in the back of your neck. We tend to forget that the back of the neck is the top of the spine and, by compressing it, the spine itself is put under pressure and distorted. To put your head and neck in the right position, look straight ahead, with your chin pulled very slightly backward. Feel as if the top of your head is attached to a piece of string that is pulling it away from your body, lengthening out your neck and spine.

Shoulders and arms

These areas are often the seat of tension in the body, and the cause of both bad posture and headaches. Look in the mirror to see if your shoulders and upper back roll forward. Perhaps they are pulled rigidly back, military fashion, pushing out your breastbone. Are they even? One shoulder is often tensed and held higher than the other, simply as a result of habitually carrying bags on one side. Check the photographs here and try to let your own shoulders drop down naturally

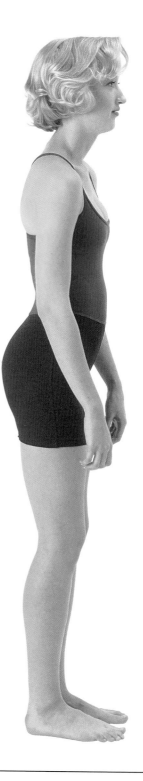

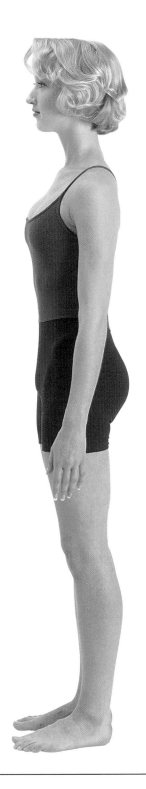

and evenly, freeing up your neck. Your arms should hang loosely, and there should be no tension in your hands and wrists. All arm movements begin in the muscles located in the middle of the back, not in the shoulders. If, during any of the exercises, you feel tension returning to your neck or shoulders, circle your shoulders a few times in each direction to loosen them up again.

Back and stomach

"Navel to spine" is the Joseph Pilates mantra. It is the first step in almost every one of his exercises for the simple reason that it is the basis of good posture. Stand sideways to the mirror. Does your lower back curve in or your stomach or bottom stick out? Now, try pushing your navel to your spine and watch the change. You should feel lengthened and gently held in. When you exercise in this position, you protect your back and strengthen your abdominal muscles.

Buttocks

As you pull your navel to your spine, you will feel your pelvis tilt very slightly upward. You need to hold this position by gently squeezing the very lowest muscles in your buttocks. This is the third element in Joseph Pilates' "girdle of strength" or "central girdle"; the others are the abdominal muscles and the Latissimus dorsi muscles in the middle of the back. Together, they hold the body in perfect alignment.

Legs and feet

Without pushing your knee too far back, your legs should be straight and elongated. If an exercise calls for a stretched leg, you should feel the stretch all the way up and through to your buttock muscles. There are two basic foot positions for all these exercises. In the first, a flexed foot forms a right angle with the leg. Don't force your toes back, as this can cause cramping, but keep them in line with the rest of your foot. In the second position, the foot is pointed. Here the foot stretches away from the ankle in a long, straight line. Again, remember not to curl your toes.

Self-assessment: the spine

PLACING THE SPINE (THE ROLLDOWN)

Joseph Pilates' technique has often – and rightly – been called "thinking exercise" for the simple reason that it is a measured, profound technique that calls for a constant awareness of each and every part of your body. In other techniques, a simple side stretch, for instance, may be just that. However, in Joseph Pilates' technique, the whole of the body is working. Before you make that stretch, you check that the effort of the movement is consolidated by the strength of the central part of the body, that there is no tension in the neck or shoulders, and that the movement originates in the proper muscles. Because posture and alignment are central to the technique, one of the most useful exercises you can do both to check and correct them is the rolldown. It will also show you how tight your hamstring muscles are.

↻ Position two
Gently drop your chin onto your chest, feeling the stretch all the way through your neck and upper back. Let the curve continue gradually so that your shoulders and upper back begin to roll forward.

↻ Position one
Stand sideways to a mirror with your feet about 18 inches (45 cm) apart. Check your posture, running through all the points on the previous pages. Your shoulders should be relaxed, dropped down into your back, with your arms hanging comfortably at your sides. Pull your navel to your spine, lift your head so that your back is relaxed and lengthened, and check that there is no arching in the small of your back.

↻ Position three

Let the curve deepen so that it reaches your lower back. Let your arms drop naturally in front of you. Now, without pushing your buttocks back – your legs should be straight, and not leaning backward – let your entire upper body hang upside down for a second or two. Try to feel the spaces between the vertebrae as you drop further, but don't strain to touch the floor if this does not happen naturally. The weight of your head will automatically stretch out your spine.

↻ Position four

Come back as slowly as possible, keeping a stretched-out feeling in your back. First, feel your buttock muscles pulling under to place your pelvis and anchor the base of your spine. Now, unroll your spine, vertebra by vertebra, keeping a tall, lengthened position, and pushing your navel to your spine. As your back unrolls, feel your shoulders drop down naturally and, last of all, place your neck and head in line with your spine. You should now be standing in a good posture, stretched and supported by the muscles of the girdle of strength. You can do the rolldown at the beginning of your exercise session at any level, just to check your posture, or if you feel at any time that you are tense or out of alignment.

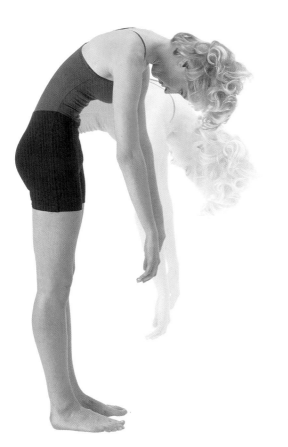

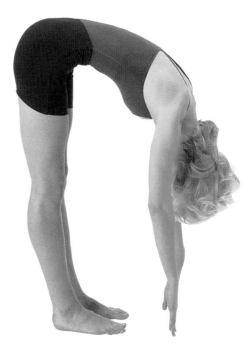

Self-assessment: the upper body

The upper body often seems to attract the stresses of everyday living. Tension can be visible and lead to problems: rigid bunched muscles, hunched shoulders, a distorted spine, poor breathing, and headaches. Joseph Pilates' technique aims to free this area, giving an elongated spine, relaxed shoulders, a long neck, and a gracefully held head.

Start by standing facing the mirror. Is your head lifted up by a long neck, or does it seem to be pushing down into your shoulders? Are your shoulders even, or is one higher? Do they roll forward, making your breastbone sink inward?

Now stand sideways and look at your reflection. Do the shoulder blades bulge out? Is your head dropping too far forward, or your chin jutting up? You should be able to trace a straight line from your ear through the shoulder down to the hips, if you are standing properly.

Try to put yourself in the correct posture using the pictures on pp. 20-21, or use the rolldown on the previous pages to help you. These two exercises will help assess your tension, and begin to free it up and improve your posture.

SHOULDER LIFT

This simple exercise will be developed later in the book. Here, use it to let your shoulders relax and drop down into their true position. Face a mirror to do this exercise. You should see a gradual change in your shoulder placement by the end of three repetitions.

Position one
Stand with good posture, and your arms relaxed by your sides. Now pull your shoulders up toward your ears as high as they will go and hold that position for a slow count of five.

Position two
Now, gently drop your shoulders down. Don't place them carefully; just let them fall. Compare how they start and finish. Adjust your posture so that your shoulders are dropped and even and the neck is long. This is the posture you want to achieve permanently.

ARM PRESSES

This exercise demonstrates where all arm movements should originate. Tension in the neck and shoulders is usually caused by using the wrong muscles to move the arms. Most people, if they lift or stretch their arms in any direction, start by moving their shoulders. In fact, arm movements should come from much lower down in the back, using the lats and lower trapezius, the muscles of the shoulder blades. This will improve posture, reduce tension, and make arm movements much more graceful.

↻ Position one

Stand in front of a mirror with your shoulders and arms relaxed, and your head held on a long neck. You are going to move your arms backward but, before your arms do anything at all, feel the muscles behind your shoulder blades (the lats) engage and pull down. You will see your shoulders drop very slightly.

↪ Position two

With your arms straight and your palms facing behind you, move the arms backward in one piece, palms out. You will feel the lats working. Stretch back, lifting your palms up, very slowly. If your shoulders start to move up, or your hands turn in, you have gone too far. If you are doing it correctly, you will feel your chest open at the same time.

Return to the starting position and repeat three to five times. Having located this feeling, try always to use the lats in this way.

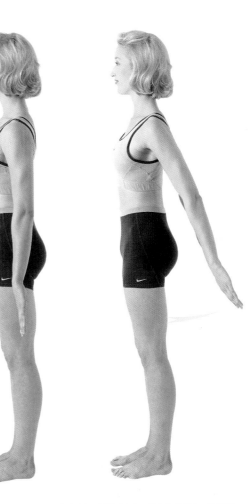

Self-assessment: the central girdle

According to Joseph Pilates, a central core of strength was the essential foundation of all exercise. He called this the "girdle of strength." It includes the Latissimus dorsi, as we have seen on the previous pages, and, most importantly, the abdomen and the buttocks. This is why, in virtually every exercise in this book, before there is any other movement the first instruction is "Take a deep breath in and, as you breathe out, draw your navel to your spine." As the muscles of this central girdle grow stronger, you are able to advance through the Joseph Pilates program in the book. Without this central core of strength, many of the later exercises would be impossible, or put a strain on the body where it would be only too likely to create problems, most notably in the back.

It is important to notice here that the effort of the exercises is always when you exhale. In some exercise techniques, including those of Joseph Pilates when taught badly, the effort is when you inhale. This causes tension and bunched muscles. By always moving when you exhale, though, you will achieve the much-desired strong but elongated body without bulging muscles.

The abdominal muscles are often weak and underused, and this can put undue strain on the back. In this technique, the abdominals are strengthened so that they are always held, not just during exercise, but throughout the day, which gives you a much more pleasing shape, as well as a stronger one! The pelvic tilt shown on p. 28 helps you to locate the abdominal muscles and use them correctly. It may seem as if very little is happening but, unless you learn to use these muscles properly, you will not be able to do the more difficult pelvic tilts later on. The surest sign of weak abdominal muscles is that they begin to bulge out with the effort. If they do this, stop immediately.

The first exercise here, the Cossack, uses the Latissimus dorsi (lats) together with the abdominals. It will help you to assess their strength as well as the flexibility of the spine.

THE COSSACK

This exercise appears in chapter four, level one. Here, it is used to check strength and flexibility. You will need to sit or stand in front of a mirror so that you can see exactly what your body is doing. Repeat it two or three times, trying to go a little further each time.

Position One

Sit or stand in front of a mirror and fold your arms loosely so that they are parallel with your breastbone. Don't grip hard with your hands as this will create tension in your neck and shoulders, which should feel relaxed and free. Your hips should be facing forward, and they do not move throughout the exercise. Breathe in and, as you breathe out, draw your lats down into your back and draw your navel to your spine.

Position two

Keeping your hips facing the mirror, turn slowly from the waist, feeling as if your body is rotating around a straight spine. Let the turn move into your upper back and, finally, your head. Don't let your shoulders tense up.

Position three

As you breathe in, come back to the starting point. Check your shoulders – they should be level and relaxed.

Position four

Repeat, turning slowly to the other side. Return to the center and repeat two or three times to each side, checking your shoulders each time you reach the central position.

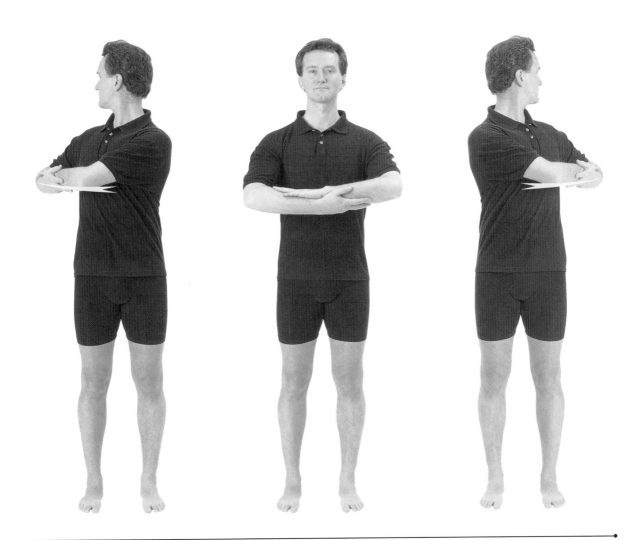

PELVIC TILT

This is the same as the very first of the pelvic tilt exercises you do in chapter four, level one. Here it is used to help you assess your posture and to locate the abdominals. Lie flat on the floor, with your legs bent at the knees, and your feet about 3 inches (7 cm) apart. Your arms should be relaxed at your sides, with no tension in your shoulders or neck. Check how much space there is between the small of your back and the floor. Ideally, it should be only a small hollow. Now, breathe in and, as you breathe out, draw your navel to your spine and you will feel the hollow reducing. It is this feeling that you want to recreate in the exercises throughout the book.

↻ Position One

Now lie with your feet up on a chair so that your knees form a right angle. The hollow in your back will be smaller than when your legs are on the floor, and your aim is to have a completely flat back in this position. Place a cushion between your thighs; this helps keep your pelvis centered throughout the exercise.

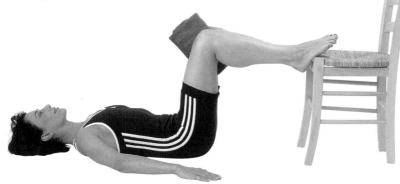

↻ Position Two

Take a deep breath and, as you breathe out, draw your navel to your spine, feeling your back flatten out along the floor. As you do this, squeeze the muscles at the very base of your buttocks; this will help you to feel a "scoop" in your abdomen. You will need this later when you do further pelvic tilts where you curl up off the floor.

SELF-HELP SUGGESTIONS

Going through this chapter, you may have noticed that some areas of your posture need work. Don't be dismayed; after all, if your posture was perfect, you wouldn't need help! Ask yourself if you can identify any of these common problems, and when you can, use the suggested exercises from chapter four to remedy them. Always do the warm-up first.

1 When you stand sideways to the mirror, does your:
➲ Stomach protrude?
➲ Bottom stick out?
➲ Lower back curve inward?
➲ Chin jut out and tilt upward?

If so, you need to work on the girdle of strength and firm up the abdominals, buttock muscles, hamstrings, and lats. Use the exercises on pp. 64, 68-69, 91, 92-93, 96, 100, 108, 109, and 133.

2 Are your shoulders stiff with tension?
➲ Do they roll forward, giving you round shoulders?
➲ Are they pulled tightly back, giving you a stiff back and neck?

If so, you need shoulder exercises. See pp. 60-61, 63, and 80.

3 Are your legs straight and do they feel elongated?
If not, use the exercises for toning the legs on pp. 70-71, 88-89, and 116-117.

4 Do the muscles above your knees droop down?
If so, practice the remedial leg exercises on pp. 72-73, 98-99, and 129.

5 When you did the rolldown on p. 22, did your lower back and hamstrings feel tight?
If so, stretch them out with the exercises on pp. 52, 100, and 133.

6 Were you able to do the pelvic tilts on p. 28 without your abdominals popping out?
If not, use the exercises from the warm-up on pp. 48-49

7 Did you remember to breathe throughout the self-assessment exercises?
If not, practice the warm-up scarf exercise on p. 50.

Remember that **STRAIN AND PAIN ARE NOT THE AIM**. Just do what you can, and you will notice a gradual but perceptible postural improvement.

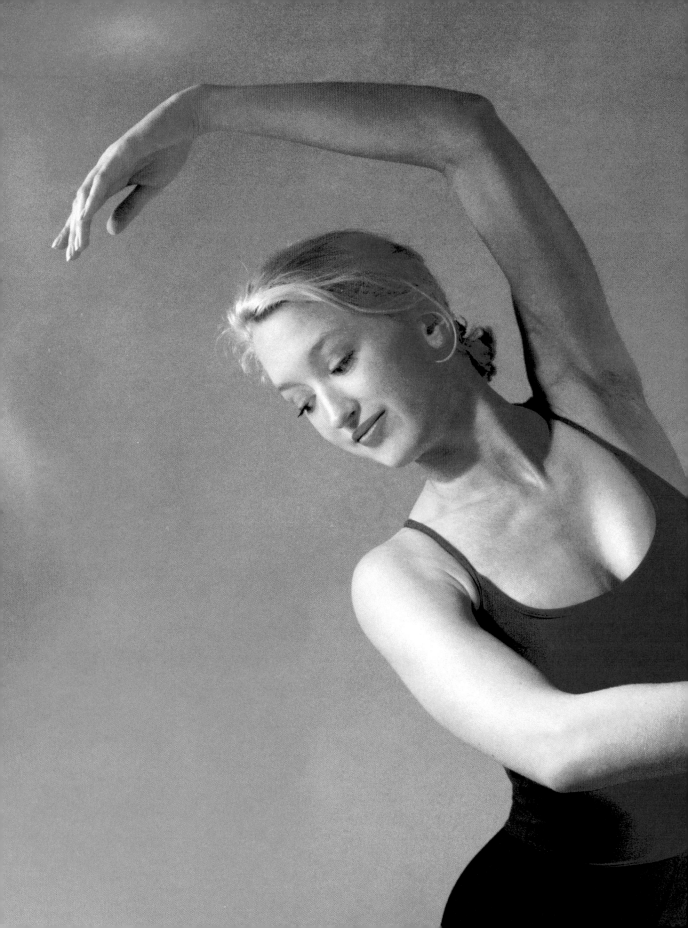

Chapter Three

A Joseph Pilates Studio

A Joseph Pilates studio is unlike any other gym. The atmosphere is calm and quiet, the music soothing, light-years away from the pumping rhythms of the aerobics studio.

Here, the benefits of the lengthening and strengthening exercises of Joseph Pilates' technique are achieved more quickly by working against the resistance of springs, pulleys, and weights. Under the guidance of an experienced teacher, posture can be perfectly realigned, while the whole body is toned and firmed. Problem areas such as flabby arms or stiff hip joints can be addressed safely, and tensions of both mind and body float gently away.

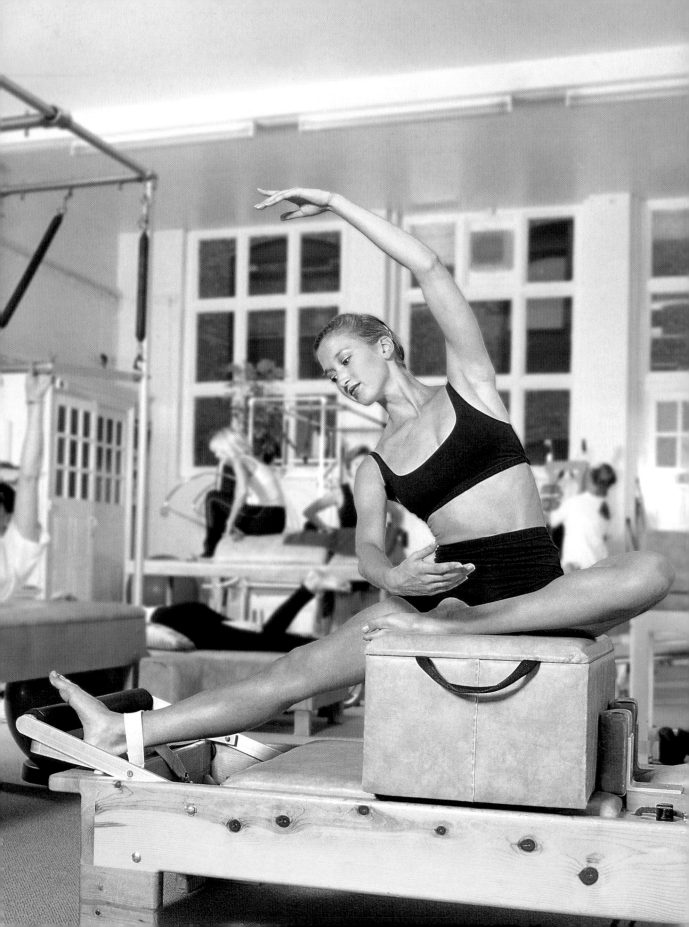

We all have different body shapes, with particular capabilities, bad habits, and ultimate potential. So, in a Joseph Pilates studio, everyone works according to a program individually designed to suit his or her own body. While people can have unrealistic expectations of any exercise system, it is certainly true that Joseph Pilates' technique can radically alter your body shape, within your particular anatomical limits.

There are two great advantages to going to a studio, even if most of your exercising takes place at home. First, when working against the resistance of the machines, you often become more aware of what a particular exercise is expecting of your body. On the plié machine, for instance, you will probably be aware of the muscles of your thighs and buttocks working more intensely than when you do pliés at home, perhaps at a deeper level within the muscle or through a greater stretch. Once you have recognized this feeling, you can incorporate the same level of intensity into your own program at home.

Second, and perhaps even more important, you get the individual attention of a teacher who will watch you throughout, adjusting your posture, demonstrating breathing and the correct movements, and giving you new exercises as you become stronger and more supple. This means you are learning the exercise properly, thus giving you more confidence on your own at home.

EXERCISING ON EQUIPMENT DESIGNED BY PILATES

The lion's share of this book, chapter four, shows you how to exercise the Joseph Pilates way at home. In this chapter, you can see how those exercises relate to the studio and what you can expect to do when you go there. All the photographs shown here were taken at Alan Herdman's studio in London, and they show only about half of the studio's equipment! If at all possible, try to go to just a few classes with a qualified instructor. Even if there is no local, fully equipped studio, there are now many "matwork" classes where Joseph Pilates' technique is taught without equipment.

SIDE STRETCH

This is a marvelous stretch for all of the muscles along your side from the hip to the rib cage. In the studio (opposite) it is performed sitting on a box on top of the plié machine. See pp. 42-43 for full, step-by-step instructions.

At home you can adapt it using a chair. The home exercise is shown in full on p. 56, and is part of the warm-up that you use to begin every exercise session.

The girdle of strength

Joseph Pilates' "girdle of strength" is centered on the abdominal muscles, and extends out to the buttocks and the lats or Latissimus dorsi, the muscles in the back that control shoulder and arm movements. The words "Breathe out, draw your navel to your spine" are repeated like a mantra in the studio. The reason for this is that the strength needed for the exercises originates in the abdominal muscles. If these muscles are not in control of a movement, then other muscles such as those in the back, neck, or shoulders attempt to carry the burden, and can be damaged. However, by using the abdominals correctly, and only as far as they are able to go at the time, you will develop strength and postural awareness. The abdominal curls or rolldowns on this page and the next three show how the muscles are strengthened and stretched in a Joseph Pilates studio.

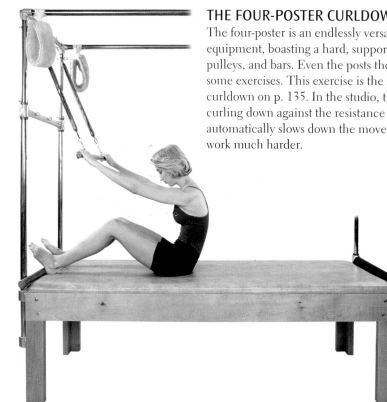

THE FOUR-POSTER CURLDOWN

The four-poster is an endlessly versatile piece of equipment, boasting a hard, supportive bed, springs, pulleys, and bars. Even the posts themselves are used for some exercises. This exercise is the studio version of the curldown on p. 135. In the studio, though, you are curling down against the resistance of two springs, which automatically slows down the movement and makes you work much harder.

↻ Position one
Begin by sitting up with your knees bent, your feet a hips' width apart, and your hands loosely holding the bar. Take a deep breath and, as you breathe out, draw your navel to your spine, letting your body curve. Your arms will begin to stretch. When they are fully extended, engage your lats, so that your shoulders pull down.

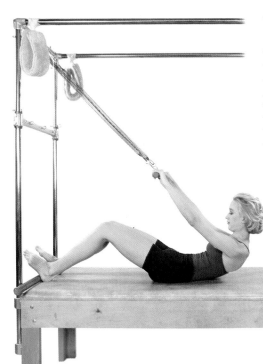

↻ Position two

Start to roll down, keeping a firm hold on your abdominal muscles. Your spine should meet the bed very slowly, so that you feel you are placing each vertebra in turn, from the base of the spine up toward your neck. Do not allow any tension to form in your arms themselves, or in your neck or shoulders. Pull the bar with your lats rather than your arms themselves; to be sure of this, you can allow your elbows to curve slightly.

↻ Position three

Your neck and head are the last parts of you to reach the bed. Keep your head curled up, until your neck lengthens. Your back should be absolutely flat against the bed, with no arching at the base of your spine. Bend your knees slightly to make sure of this. When you are flat against the bed, take a long breath in and curve slowly back up again.

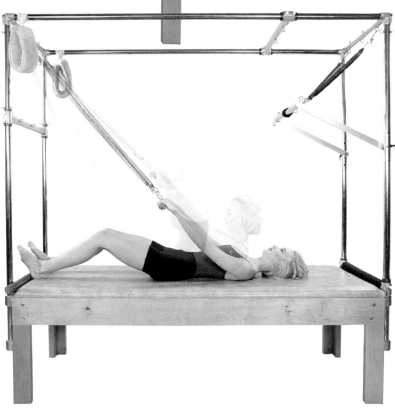

The abdominals

ABDOMINAL CURLS ON A BOX

This is a much more advanced abdominals exercise. It takes place on the plié machine, which has a box placed on top of it to form a seat, while the feet are tucked under a strap. In this exercise, you do not work against the resistance of springs, but you do hold a pole that keeps your arms stretched and level throughout. This is a very hard exercise and one that requires real strength in the abdominal muscles and a good deal of postural awareness.

⮑ Position one

Begin by sitting on the box, with your legs straight and your feet sufficiently flexed to keep the strap in place. Sit very tall on the box, pulling up out of your hips so that your buttocks and legs are working. Making sure that your back stays absolutely straight, with your neck in line with your spine, raise your arms, bringing the pole above your head. There should be no tension in your shoulders or neck; you should be able to turn your head freely from side to side. Take a deep breath in.

⮑ Position two

As you breathe out, draw your navel to your spine and start to curl your back down so that your abdominal muscles scoop, and your head and shoulders curve gently toward your body. At the same time, lower your arms gradually until they are stretched out in front of you.

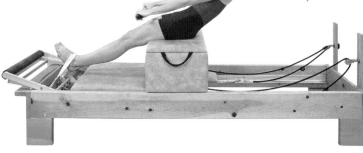

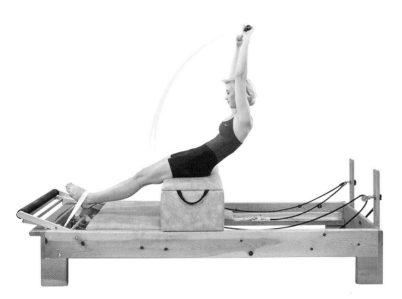

↻ Position three

Holding the curve – don't let your abdominal muscles pop out during the next movement – raise the pole above your head until your arms are stretched up toward the ceiling again. Don't let any tension form in your neck or shoulders, or let the effort go into the small of your back.

↻ Position four

Keeping the same shape in your body, bring the pole down in front of you, until you are in the same position as position 2.

↻ Position five

Roll up, vertebra by vertebra, until you are sitting in the same position as position 1, with your arms holding the pole above your head. Take a deep breath and check where you feel any tension. The work of this exercise should take place only in your abdominals. If you feel the effort anywhere else, it means your abdominal muscles are not yet strong enough for this very strenuous exercise.

The lats and torso

The "lats" or Latissimus dorsi, are the uppermost section of Joseph Pilates' "girdle of strength," and are frequently forgotten by most of us. The lats are the muscles behind the shoulder blades, and should form the source of all arm and shoulder movement. Most people use the shoulders themselves instead of the lats when they move their arms. This results in tension in the neck and shoulders, often with accompanying tension headaches. Together with strong abdominal muscles, proper use of the lats virtually guarantees good posture. They are muscles that are definitely worth remembering and bringing back into use.

The exercises shown here engage the lats and the trapezius muscles above them, and stretch out the upper torso. When many of us sit with hunched posture and rounded shoulders, this stretching inevitably brings a great feeling of release and freedom in the upper body.

LOCATING THE LATS

This is a good exercise for locating the lats and learning how to use them properly. It relates to the one on p. 62. Ideally, you should do them both in front of a mirror. This enables you to see what your shoulders are doing – if you're doing it properly, they should be doing nothing! The work takes place in the back so, as the bar raises and lowers, you shouldn't be able to see any movement at all in your shoulder itself.

Position one
Sit squarely, with your knees together, your shoulders dropped down into your back, and your spine straight. Breathe in and, as you breathe out, draw your navel toward your spine. Holding the bar lightly with your fingertips, lower it by drawing down your lats.

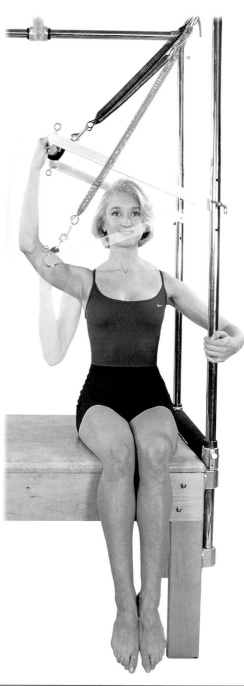

Position two
Allow the bar to return to the starting position. Feel the movement in your lats only, and keep your shoulders quite still.

Stretching out the upper torso

This is the studio version of the exercise on pp. 122-123.
Try to stretch your upper body without tensing your
shoulders and, in position two, keep your arms touching
the bed for as long as you can, to release the shoulder
joint and free up your back. The sensation of the stretch is
wonderfully elongating.

Position one
Lie on your back with your knees raised and the
entire length of your spine pressed into the bed.
Stretch out your arms to hold the bar, without
tension. Breathe in and, as you breathe out,
press your navel further into the bed, and start
to draw the bar down toward you.

Position two
As your upper arms reach the bed, start to circle your
elbows out so that the bar goes further away from your
body. Keep your upper arms in contact with the bed for
as long as possible. When your arms cannot stay on the
bed any longer, breathe out and stretch them out behind
your head, still keeping your spine flat on the bed.
Breathe in, and return to position two. Breathe out, and
return to the starting position.

The arms and upper body

These exercises are all slow, small, and deceptively simple. The upper torso exercises use the lats and the trapezius muscles while opening up and releasing the chest. The arm exercises are very similar to those on pp. 74-75 but, as the body is raised off the ground on a piece of equipment called the barrel, it gives the arms a greater stretch.

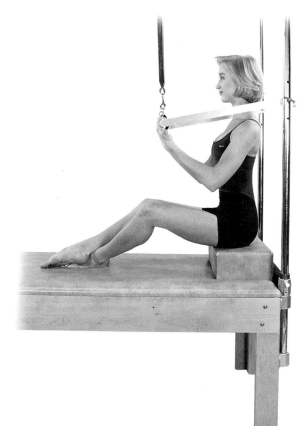

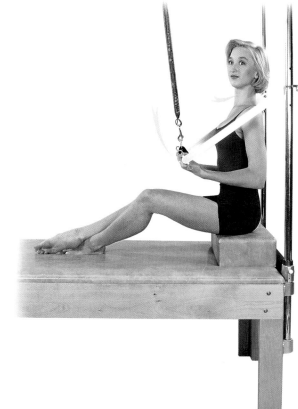

UPPER TORSO

⌒ Position one
Sitting very tall on a small box, with your legs stretched out and crossed at the ankles, place your fingertips loosely on the bar. Your head should be in line with a long straight spine and there should be no tension anywhere in your body.

⌒ Position two
Breathe in and, as you breathe out, draw the bar down very slowly, feeling your chest open, your neck lengthen, and your head lift and turn toward your left shoulder. Return to the center and alternate right and left.

TRICEPS EXERCISE

The triceps are the muscles in the back of your upper arms and this exercise is great for flabby upper arms.

Position one

Lie with your knees bent and your back flat against the barrel. Check that there is no arch in the small of your back. Hold the weight in both hands so that it drops down toward your chest.

Position two

Breathe in and, as you breathe out, draw your navel to your spine and, in one smooth movement, lift the weight over your head as far as you can. Breathe in and return to the starting position.

ARM OPENINGS

Here, you use two weights of up to 2 pounds (1 kg) each. This exercise tones the arm muscles and opens up the back and chest and releases the shoulder joints.

Position one

Lie on the barrel with your knees raised, your entire spine on the barrel, and your arms in a wide curve, your hands meeting above your chest. Feel as if you are holding a beach ball within the curve of your arms.

Position two

Breathe in and, as you breath out, draw your navel to your spine and open your arms outward, still retaining the curve. Return to the starting position.

USING ARM WEIGHTS

These exercises relate directly to those in chapter four. All the arm exercises given later start off without weights, because you add them only when you have built up some strength. You can substitute cans of beans for the weights, but working against any form of weight is beneficial, especially as we age. Weight work can actually prevent osteoporosis in menopausal and post-menopausal women. Use weights of up to 2 pounds (1 kg).

SIDE STRETCHES

This advanced exercise requires a great deal of strength and postural awareness. It stretches out both sides of the body in turn and has a very graceful, dancerlike feeling to it. Again, it uses a box on the plié machine and the position is secured by the foot strap, and a lot of control.

➲ Position one

Sit on the box with your right foot tucked under the strap and your left leg bent and resting on the box. Your back should be completely straight, with your head lifted and in line with your spine. Your right arm is raised in a graceful curve, and your left arm is curved in front of your body.

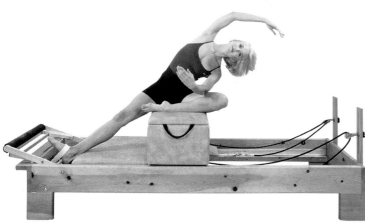

↻ Position two

Take a deep breath in and, as you breathe out, draw your navel to your spine and bend smoothly over to the left. Your arms and legs should remain in exactly the same relationship to your body as in position one.

➲ Position three

Now reverse your arms so that your left is extended in a curve away from your body and your right is curved in front.

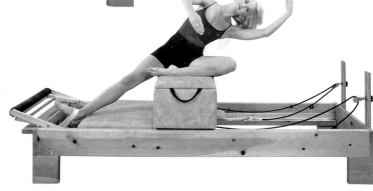

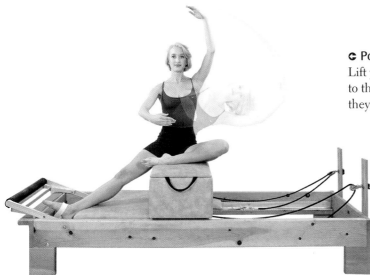

c Position four

Lift your body in one smooth movement back to the starting position, keeping your arms as they were in position three.

⊃ Position five

Take another breath and, as you breathe out, bend the other way so that your left arm is curving down toward your right foot. Keep drawing your navel to your spine.

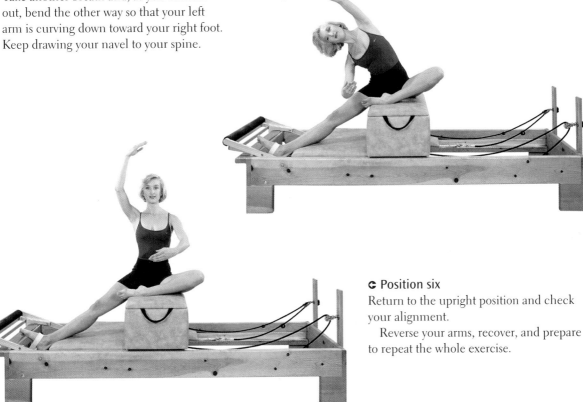

c Position six

Return to the upright position and check your alignment.

Reverse your arms, recover, and prepare to repeat the whole exercise.

Pliés

Pliés are one of the fundamental ballet exercises. Though they may look like simple knee bends, they are actually much more complex. When performed correctly, the plié uses most of the body. Because they are complex movements, they are not brought into the home routine until level three (pp. 130-131), by which time you will have greater body awareness and will be able to focus on several areas at the same time. In the studio, you do them on the plié machine, which helps in various ways. First, because you are lying down, your spine is straight and you are less prone to bad posture and injury. Second, working against springs is harder and enables you to become aware of the muscles in the abdominals, legs, and buttocks that you should be using. As you can add up to four springs for resistance, the work is more intense and your muscles become toned up faster.

PLIÉS FIRST POSITION
↻ Position one
Begin with the bed of the plié machine close to the footrest. Place your feet so that your your toes are on the footrest and your heels are together, forming a V-shape. This position for the feet is called "turned out," which means that your whole leg follows the same direction. Without exaggerating the position, your knees should be facing slightly outward and your legs should feel the turnout all the way from your hip socket downward. Make sure your back and neck are in a long straight line, and your arms and shoulders are relaxed at your sides.

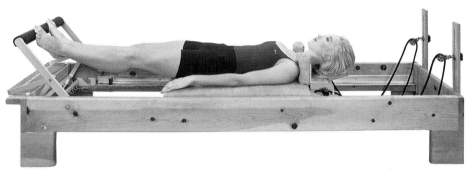

⟳ Position two
Breathe in, breathe out, draw your navel to your spine, and push away from the footrest until your legs are straight. As you push, feel the turnout strongly in your thighs and buttocks. The muscles should feel as if they are wrapping around – imagine your inner thigh trying to face upward. Breathe in; return to position one.

PLIÉS SECOND POSITION
⟳ Position one
This time, position your feet so that your heels are on the outside edges of the footrest. With your knees dropping out to the sides, you should feel a sense of openness in your hip socket. Check your spinal alignment before you move on to the next stage.

⟳ Position two
Breathe in and, as you breathe out, draw your navel to your spine and push away from the footrest until your legs are straight. Feel the turnout. Breathe in to return to position 1. Repeat each position 10 times.

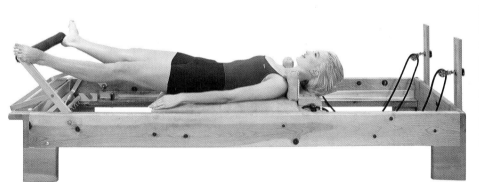

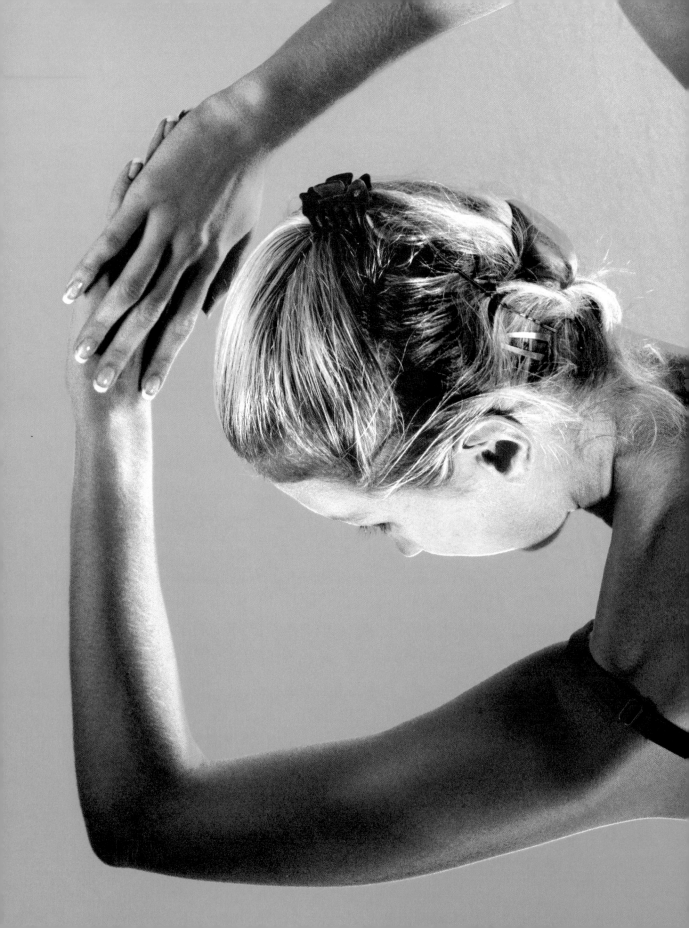

Chapter Four

Joseph Pilates' Workout

This workout is the safest, most thorough way to achieve the shape you've always wanted. You will look and feel better within weeks and, on completion, have a dancer's strong, lean, flexible physique.

The program's golden rule is: Don't rush it. Always warm up before you exercise; this trains your body's memory to use the proper muscles every time. Don't be tempted to advance to another level until you have mastered the current one or you may strain your muscles and joints. Each level is designed to strengthen your body as an integrated whole. Plan to exercise three times a week in a tranquil environment. Feel your body changing – and enjoy it.

The warm-up session

A Joseph Pilates warm-up is quite different from other warm-ups. Because the exercises are so precise, it is vital to be sure you are moving correctly, and the warm-up helps you to locate, isolate, and develop all of the key areas to be used in the exercises to come.

The same warm-up applies to all three levels, because all three use the same muscles, though with varying degrees of difficulty and complexity. However, there is another reason for the warm-up repetition.

As every dancer knows, the body, not just the mind, has a memory, and by repeating these movements regularly, they will inform not only your exercise session, but every single movement of your daily life.

YOU WILL NEED

Essentials

- *Comfortable clothing*
- *A soft carpet, towel, or yoga mat to lie on*
- *A long scarf*
- *A medium-sized towel*
- *Firm cushions of various sizes*
- *A chair or stool (your knees must bend at 90° when seated on it)*
- *An item of household furniture that supports your weight, such as a table or door frame*

Extras

- *Hand-held weights, either 2-pound (1-kg) dumbbells or ordinary food cans*
- *Strap-on 2-pound (1-kg) leg weights*
- *A lightweight pole or broom handle*

BREATHING

Though this exercise may suggest that little is happening, it is fundamental. Because deep rhythmic breathing is so important and, indeed, shapes all of the exercises, it is vital to start by establishing proper breathing. You may find that slow classical music will help keep your breathing steady and rhythmic. Or, if you prefer, set the pace by your own breath.

☋ Position one

Lie on your back, with your feet up on a chair, and your knees forming a right angle. Make sure you lie straight, with no tension in your neck and shoulders. Place a bolster or rolled-up towel between your knees. Make a diamond shape with your hands over the abdominal muscles, and rest your head on a book.

➲ Position two

Now breathe very slowly and deeply, feeling each breath reach the abdominal area so that your hands rise and fall with the breath. Try to create a constant, slow, deep rhythm. This is how you need to breathe throughout the exercises. Repeat for 10 slow, deep breaths.

THE SCOOP

This is a continuation of the previous exercise and transforms the breathing into a movement.

↻ Lie on the floor, with your spine lengthened, the small of your back touching the floor, and your neck and shoulders relaxed. Place a bolster or rolled-up towel between your knees.

Breathe in and, as you breathe out, draw your navel to your spine and squeeze your low buttock muscles so that the abdominal muscles are scooped into a spoon shape. Do this 10 times, trying to extend the scoop further each time.

THE SCOOP

The scoop teaches the basis of all pelvic tilt exercises and you can use it to feel these muscles in their entirety. The more of the abdominal muscles that you can engage, the better – these muscles almost reach the pelvic area and can be scooped up the whole way.

THE SCARF

This is another exercise to help achieve the proper breathing you need for Joseph Pilates' technique. Keep the scarf taut – but not tight – throughout, and it will help you focus on your breathing.

➲ Position one

Stand, or sit on a chair or stool so that your knees form a right angle when your feet are flat on the floor. Your toes should point straight forward. Take a scarf and wrap it around your upper body so that it covers the whole depth of your ribs. Cross it in front of you and hold one end in each hand.

➤ Position two

Take a deep breath in and fill your lungs with air, keeping your lats pulled down into your back. The scarf will help you to feel how far your lungs expand; you should be able to feel your back widen as well as your chest, if you are breathing properly.

➲ Position three

Breathe out and feel your body empty of air, keeping the scarf taut. Repeat for 10 breaths, trying to expand your lungs a little further each time.

DOMING

Most people hardly use the muscles in their feet, and this often results in inflexibility. This exercise shows you how to release "frozen" feet – keep the image of a cat drawing in its claws in your mind and you'll have the right idea! It is also a good exercise for getting your foot working properly again if you have had an injury. You should do it with bare feet.

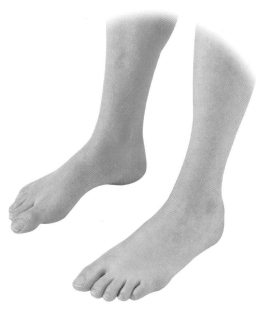

∩ Position one
Sit on a chair, with your knees bent at right angles and your feet flat on the floor a hips' width apart.

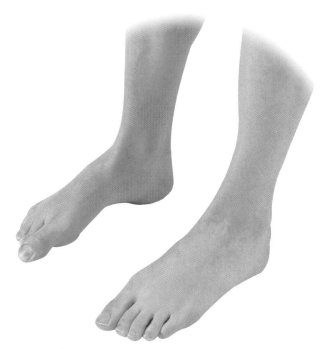

∩ Position two
Draw your toes back against the floor so that your instep lifts but your heel stays firmly on the floor. Don't expect a big movement, especially at first. Do not let your toes curl under. Hold the lift for a few seconds, before straightening your toes and returning to the starting postion. Repeat 10 times.

FOOT MASSAGE

After doming, you can give yourself a foot massage. This can be very relaxing, especially if you are prone to cramps. Start by gently stroking your entire foot. Then apply a firmer pressure by circling your thumbs all over the sole. Finally, apply the same pressure on top of your foot between each of your toes. Pull each toe out from its base, stretching it gently and smoothly.

Releasing the back and neck

The following two exercises release tension stored in the back and the neck. These are problem areas for many people who can often be unaware that any such tension exists. Once you have freed up the back and the neck, your posture will be improved instantly.

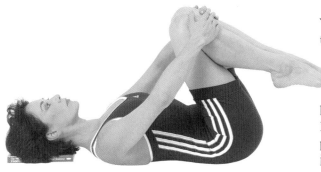

KNEE TO CHEST
You will feel the lower vertebrae open up as you do this exercise.

☾ Position one
Lie on your back so that your entire spine is touching the floor. Bend and lift your knees, keeping them slightly apart, in line with your hips. Draw your navel gently to your spine and hold this position throughout the exercise. Place your hands just below, not on, your knees.

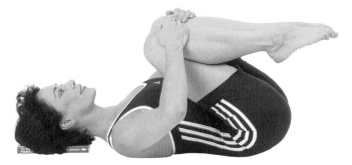

➲ Position two
Breathe in and, as you breathe out, gently draw your knees to your chest, keeping your arms wide. Make sure your entire spine remains on the floor. Feel your back and chest open out as you do this.

☾ Position three
Breathe in and, on the next exhale, draw your right leg to your chest. Release and, on the next exhale, draw your left leg to your chest. Repeat in the same sequence – right, then left, then knees together – 10 times.

HIP ROLLS – BEGINNERS

This is the first of the hip rolls – you will find later versions throughout the book. In this first stage, concentrate on releasing your lower back and feeling the stretch across your abdomen.

↺ Position one

Lie on your back, with your knees bent and pointing to the ceiling, and your feet together. Put your hands on your abdominals to help you feel them stretch. Keep your back and neck long and relaxed.

IMPORTANT

- *Do not try to force your knees too far toward the floor, or your back and buttocks will lift up.*
- *Always keep your knees exactly aligned.*
- *Roll straight to the side, with no twisting.*

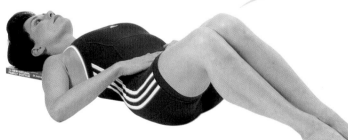

↻ Position two

Breathe in and, as you breathe out, roll your knees to one side, keeping your buttocks glued to the floor and your knees together. You will not be able to go very far but you should still feel a strong stretch across your abdominals.

↺ Position three

Breathe in to return to the center and check your position. Breathe out, and repeat on the other side. Alternate, 10 rolls to each side.

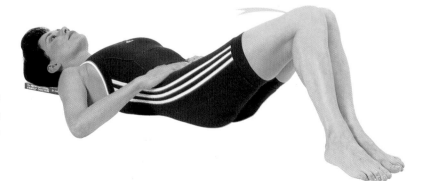

Releasing the upper body

These exercises are very good for anyone who has a tendency to store tension in the shoulders, neck, or back. They release the upper body and help to get the lats working properly, the muscles that you should be using to initiate arm movements, rather than your shoulders.

SHOULDER SHRUGS

In this exercise you can lift your shoulders rather than pull them down into the back.

↺ Position one

Sit on a chair in front of a mirror, with your feet flat on the floor and facing forward. If you have a bolster cushion, stand this on its end between your knees to help stabilize your pelvis. Let your arms hang down relaxed at your sides.

↻ Position two

Now, breathe in and lift up your shoulders toward your ears.

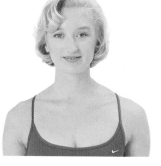

↺ Position three

As you breathe out, lower your shoulders and gently stretch your hands down to the floor. Rotate your arms inward and stretch them behind you – but not too far. If you are doing it properly, this will open up your chest and strengthen the muscles below your shoulder blades. Repeat 10 times.

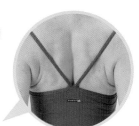

As you draw your arms back, feel your lats pulling down and squeezing together.

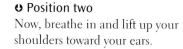

NOSE FIGURE 8

The movement involved in this exercise is so small that it looks almost as though nothing is happening but it actually involves a great deal of concentration. While your mind is involved in controlling the movement, the back of your neck relaxes without your noticing.

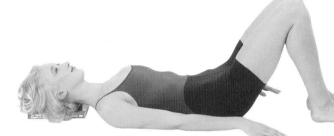

↺ Position one

Lie on your back, with your spine stretched out along the floor, and your knees bent. Place your arms down by your sides, draw your navel gently toward your spine, and squeeze your lower buttock muscles. Hold this position throughout.

↻ Position two

Focus all of your attention on the tip of your nose and make it trace a figure eight in the air. This is only a tiny movement; your face does not turn from side to side. Do 10 figure eights in one direction, then reverse it and do 10 more. You may find that closing your eyes helps you focus on the movement.

SIDE STRETCHES – BEGINNERS

This is the first of two side-stretching exercises. This one concentrates on the area from the waist to the elbows. The second one, in which you are standing, takes the stretch down through the hips too.

U Positions two and three

Take a deep breath in and, as you breathe out, turn your head to the right and gently stretch your left side, elbow first, up to the ceiling and then dipping down toward the floor in a big curve. Breathe in to return to the starting position and repeat 10 times on each side.

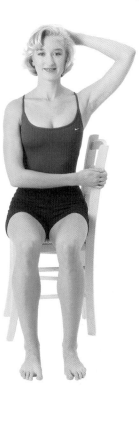

↻ Position one

Sit on a straight chair with your left side against its back. Place your right hand on the chair back so that your arm crosses in front of your body. Put your left hand behind your head. Make sure your body is square and facing forward, with your knees a hips' width apart and the toes pointing forward.

SIDE STRETCHES – ELEMENTARY

In this second side stretch, this time in the standing position, you take the stretch further. The greater the distance between you and your support, the further you will be able to stretch.

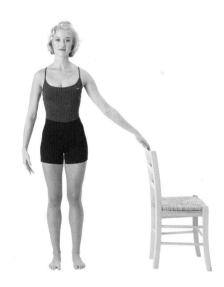

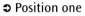
↪ Position one
Stand, holding on to a well-anchored chair or a door frame, about a foot away from it. Your feet should be apart, your shoulders dropped, with no tension in your upper body.

↩↪ Position two
Breathe in and, as you breathe out, stretch away from the chair, letting your outer arm describe a wide circle until your hand reaches back over your head. Feel the stretch all the way through your side. Return to the starting position and repeat 10 times on each side.

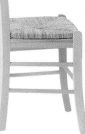

CHECK BOX

- *Keep your feet slightly apart and flat on the floor throughout.*
- *Don't let your body twist – your hips should face squarely to the front throughout.*
- *Keep your upper body free from tension – arms, shoulders, and neck should be open and free.*

Joseph Pilates' Workout: level one

Level one is undoubtedly the most important stage of your program. It is here that you learn how to use your body correctly, and the new way of moving that you will master now is the basis of all the more complex exercises to come.

For this reason alone, don't hurry to move on. By learning to move each part of your body with precision, you will tone and strengthen your muscles as well as improving your posture.

Right from the start, you should establish your exercise routine as a time for quiet concentration. Turn off the telephone, or put on the answering machine. Find yourself a warm, comfortable space, and put on some quiet classical music. This will help you to slow down. Above all, remember that these exercises are to be done rhythmically and very slowly.

Your goals for level one

- Concentrate on your alignment and posture above all
- If you feel you are standing or sitting incorrectly or you can feel muscles tensing up, repeat the posture exercises on pp. 20-28 until you feel that your placement is as it should be.
- Don't rush any of the exercises, even if they feel easy.
- Concentrate instead on making each one precise and controlled.
- Keep your awareness on your entire body, and don't let any one part take over.
- Always check that your entire body is in the correct position, relaxed and lengthened.
- Focus on your breathing – it should be deep, slow, and rhythmical, with all the effort performed when you exhale.

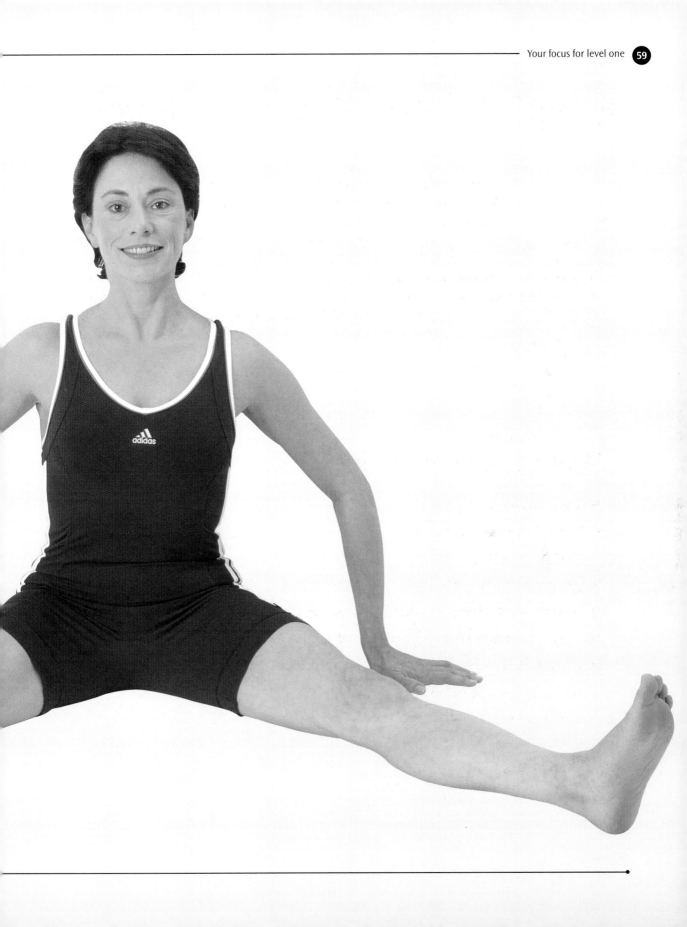

Releasing the upper body

These exercises work on the posture. The upper body is one of the three fundamental areas to be strengthened in Joseph Pilates' technique (the others are the abdominals and the buttocks) and it centers on the lats and trapezius, the muscles of the back. These should also be the source of all your arm movements, rather than your shoulders themselves. As the lats and trapezius become strengthened, posture naturally improves with the shoulders dropping down and becoming more relaxed, the chest and the rib cage opening, and the neck and head held properly and without tension.

OPENINGS – BEGINNERS

Keep your upper arms glued to your sides in this exercise for a wonderful feeling of opening and relaxation in your upper body.

↻ Position one

Sit on a chair or support at the right height for your knees to bend at a 90° angle. Your feet should be flat on the floor, a hips' width apart, with your toes pointing straight ahead. There should be no tension in your neck or shoulders. Hold your upper arms firmly against your sides, bending them at the elbows so they are at a 90° angle, with the palms up.

↺ Position two

Breathe in and put your palms out to the sides so they make a semicircle around your body, keeping your upper arms by your sides.

As you breathe out, return to the starting position, with your fingers pointing forward. Repeat 10 times.

OPENINGS – ELEMENTARY

Let your arms feel as if they are carrying your breath around your body in this exercise.

THINK TALL

To get the most out of this exercise, sit with a long, straight spine. Feel your neck as a natural extension of your spine, with your head balanced and lifted. It helps to imagine that a piece of string is attached to your head, pulling it gently upward.

➲ Position one

Sit in the same position as for the previous exercise, this time with your palms facing down.

➲ Position two

Breathe in and move your arms out to the sides, rotating them as before.

This time, when they have rotated as far as they will go, release them from your body so that your hands reach slightly outward – only a very small gap should open up.

Breathe out to return to the starting position. Repeat 10 times.

Strengthening the back

In the studio, a series of exercises is performed using the resistance of springs to help isolate the muscles around the shoulders and thus use them more effectively. You can do the same exercises at home, however, without equipment. Just make sure you feel the movement in your back first; draw the muscles down before you begin to move your arm. Here is the first of the upper back exercises.

UPPER BACK RELEASE – BEGINNERS
This is a small movement. Do it slowly and precisely for maximum effect.

➲ Position one
Sit on a chair or stool close to the wall, with your feet firmly on the floor and your knees forming a right angle. Bend your arm at the elbow to make a right angle and place the back of your hand and your lower arm flat against the wall.

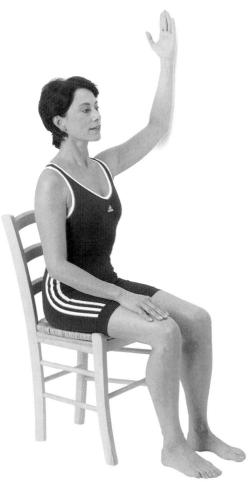

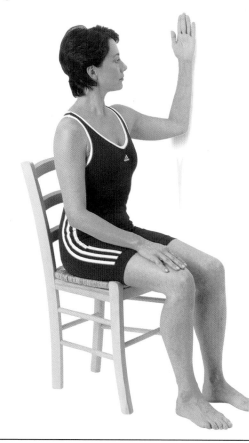

↺ Position two
Breathe in and, as you breathe out, draw your navel toward your spine and draw your shoulder blades downward. Let this movement in your shoulder blades draw your arm downward, still against the wall. The movement is only one of a few inches, but you should feel the muscles working deep inside your back. Breathe in to return to the starting position, and repeat 10 times on each side.

THE COSSACK

This exercise was given as an aid to self-assessment on p. 26. Now you do it sitting down. In all these exercises, your navel is held gently against your spine, with your back straight, and your shoulders and neck relaxed. The movement begins by drawing down your lats, the muscles below your shoulder blades, so you should feel your shoulders themselves drop as you move.

CHECKLIST

■ *Check that your shoulders are down and level each time you return to center.*
■ *Keep your feet firmly on the floor.*
■ *Make sure your hands stay loose throughout.*
■ *Don't let your hips turn to the sides as you move.*
■ *Make sure there is no tension in your neck.*

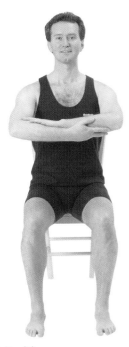

ᴖ Position one

Sit on a stool with your feet flat on the floor, and toes pointing forward. Fold your arms loosely, parallel with your sternum. Don't grip on or hold any tension in them. Your hips should face forward and stay in this position throughout the exercise. Draw your navel to your spine and hold it firmly throughout the exercise. Draw down the lats toward the base of your spine.

ᴄ Position two

Breathe in deeply and, as you breathe out, begin to turn from the waist, but keep your hips facing squarely to the front. Take the turn into your upper back, and let your head follow last.

Breathe in and come back to the starting position. As you breathe out, turn to the other side, then repeat 10 turns on each side in a smooth, continuous movement.

Isolating the abdominals

This first exercise is the same as the one shown earlier in the book that helped you assess your posture. Here it is used as an exercise in its own right and an introduction to a series of exercises in which you work on the movement that initiates all the pelvic tilts.

CHECKLIST

- *Make sure you breathe correctly – the breathing is a vital part of this exercise.*
- *Think of your abdominal muscles helping to curve your spine. Ideally, your back should become as sinuous as a snake!*
- *Don't let any tension get into your shoulders, chest, or neck. If they start to tense, you are coming too far off the floor.*
- *Always begin by drawing down your navel and engaging your low buttock muscles for a moment before you start to move off the floor.*
- *The more slowly you do these pelvic tilts, the more effective they are.*

PELVIC TILTS – BEGINNERS ENGAGING

You can use this exercise to help you isolate the abdominal muscles.

➲ Position one

Lie on your back with your feet raised on a box or a straight chair so that your knees form a right angle. Put a cushion between your thighs – this is not to squeeze, but to keep the pelvis centered through the exercise.

↻ Position two

Take a deep breath, then, as you breathe out, draw your navel down toward your spine, feeling it flatten out along the floor. At the same time, squeeze the muscles at the very base of your buttocks, but try to avoid squeezing the hamstrings in your thighs. Don't lift off the floor at all. Breathe in and return to the starting position. Repeat this exercise 10 times.

PELVIC TILTS ELEMENTARY – CURLING UP

Go on to this exercise only when you have located exactly which muscles you should be using, and always do stage one first as a reminder. Don't try to curl up too high at this stage. Staying in control is more important than height.

⊃ Position one

Lie in exactly the same position as for the previous exercise. Breathe in deeply and, as you breathe out, draw your navel to your spine and squeeze your lowest buttock muscles.

↻ Position two

This time you let the squeeze continue so that it draws your body up, tightening your inner thighs and raising your body, vertebra by vertebra, in an arc from the floor. At the top, breathe in and curl down slowly. Repeat 10 times.

Strengthening the abdominals

Sit-ups demand a great deal of strength in the abdominal muscles if they are not to put a strain on the back. Unfortunately, many gyms and classes use sit-ups, often with a lot of repetitions, as a basic exercise, without giving proper instruction on how to do them without injury to the back and with the emphasis on how far you get up off the floor. In fact, in a good sit-up with strongly held abdominals, you come off the floor only a little way, but your abdominals curve in rather than popping out.

CHECKLIST

- *Don't expect to get your shoulders off the floor at first. In time, you will be able to get your lats off the floor but the most important factor here is that you work only your abdominals and don't let your back take any strain at all.*
- *If you feel any strain in your back, stop.*
- *Don't drop your chin onto your chest. Your body comes up in a curved unit.*

SIT-UPS – BEGINNERS
➲ Position one

Lie on your back with your knees raised and a pad or book to support your head and shoulders. Put a cushion between your knees, too, not to squeeze during the exercise, but simply to stabilize the pelvis and keep your hips square. Your upper body should be open and relaxed – check for any tension before you begin. Place your hands on the top of your thighs.

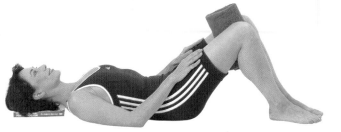

↻ Position two

Breathe in and, as you breathe out, draw your navel to your spine and squeeze your low buttock muscles together. Slowly walk your fingers up your thighs toward your knees, letting your head and shoulders curl up off the floor as they get higher. Keep your navel pressed to your spine. If it starts to pop out, you have come up too far.

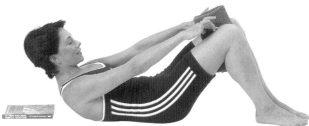

➲ Position three

At the top, breathe in and, as you breathe out, draw in your stomach muscles and roll slowly back down to the floor, sliding your fingers back down your legs.

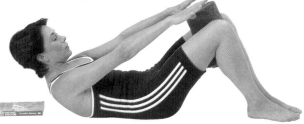

↻ Position four

When you are back in the starting position, take a deep breath and rest. Work up to 10 repeats.

OBLIQUE SIT-UPS – BEGINNERS

Oblique sit-ups work the abdominal muscles at the sides that are just as important as those at the front. In this first exercise, don't expect to come a long way off the floor. Concentrate on becoming aware of where your oblique abdominals are.

↺ Position one

Lie on your back, with your raised and a cushion betwee in the previous exercise. Pu feet flat on the floor and you hand behind your head. Your right arm stays flat on the floor at your side, with the palm facing down.

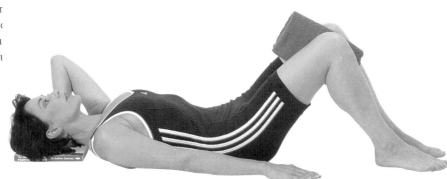

↻ Position two

Breathe in and, as you breathe out, draw your navel to your spine and engage the muscles at the base of your buttocks. Now, using your left hand to support your head, curve diagonally, aiming your left elbow and shoulder toward your right knee. At the same time, stretch your right hand down in the direction of your feet.

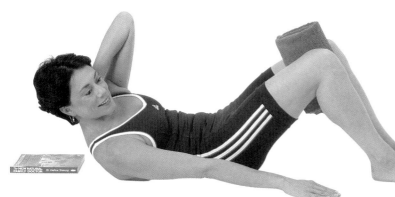

↺ Position three

Breathe in and, breathing out, draw back to the starting position. Work up to 10 sit-ups on each side.

Strengthening the central girdle

This is the first of a series of exercises that work on strengthening the abdominal muscles and correcting the alignment of the pelvis and spine. The strength of this central girdle of the body is essential to good posture and the strength of the body as a whole. It is also a vital protection for the back. Weak abdominal muscles and poor alignment will inevitably put a strain on the back and leave it open to injury.

Proper breathing helps to strengthen and protect the muscles of the back. Although your natural inclination may be to pull your stomach in as you breathe in – many people have this tendency when they try to "stand up straight" – you should be doing the opposite. So, as you are breathing out, draw your abdominal muscles to your spine, and make the effort of the movement.

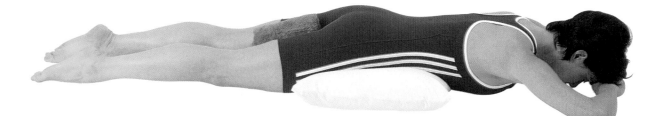

BUTTOCK SQUEEZE

This exercise is very good for locating and beginning to use the lower part of Joseph Pilates' "girdle of strength" – you quite literally begin to get a grip on the abdominals and the muscles at the base of your buttocks.

CHECKLIST

- *Don't let the small of the back curve in as you squeeze the cushion – keep your navel drawn toward your spine.*
- *Your upper body should be free – don't let your neck or shoulders tense up with effort.*
- *Your lower legs and feet should be relaxed – the muscles in the lowest part of your buttocks are doing the work.*

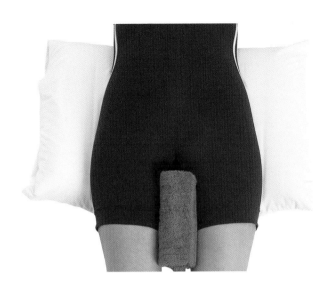

↷ Position one
Lie face down with a pillow to support your abdomen and a small cushion between your thighs. You can lie on the floor or, ideally, a hard bed, so that your feet hang just over the edge. Place your head on your hands, turning it to one side if you prefer. Breathe in.

↷ Position two
As you breathe out, draw your navel to your spine and, at the same time, squeeze the cushion between your thighs using the muscles at the very base of your buttocks. Don't engage your hamstrings or the rest of your buttock muscles. Just try to isolate this one set of muscles. Release, and repeat 10 times.

↻ Rest position
After you have finished the buttock squeeze, this rest position is very good for getting rid of any strain you might feel.

From the position of the previous exercise, draw your body back so that your bottom is sitting on your heels. At first it is unlikely that you'll reach your heels, but just get as close as you can. Leave your arms outstretched on the bed and feel a long stretch all the way through your back. Hold this position for about two minutes and let your back feel as if it is ironing itself out.

A BIGGER STRETCH

As you become looser, you will find that you can manage to sit on your heels. To help you stretch, ask a friend to put one hand at the top of your back and the other in the small of your back, and push the hands apart gently. This extends the stretch, and feels wonderful!

Toning the legs

These exercises are the first in a series that stretch and strengthen the leg muscles from the buttocks right down to the feet. The alignment of the body is very important if you want the legs to work properly, so many of these exercises are performed on your side with your back against the wall – ensuring that shoulders and hips stay square. It is also vital that your leg is in the correct position before you begin any of the exercises; if you can set up a mirror, it's a good idea to check it to make sure you're parallel, or turned out.

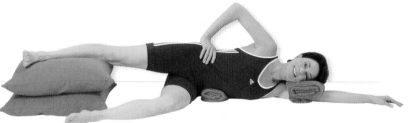

A FLAT BACK

In this exercise, it is very important to keep your back absolutely flat against the wall, with your hips facing directly forward. This will keep your legs parallel.

OUTER THIGHS – BEGINNERS

This exercise creates a very pleasing hollow in the outer thigh rather than that all-too-common bulge.

↻ Position one

Lie on your side with your back flat against a wall. Let your lower arm stretch out, and place a pillow or towel folded double between this arm and your head. It is also a good idea to place a small cushion or folded towel beneath your waist as this gives support and reminds you not to let your waist fall in. Bend your lower leg and place your upper leg on a large, firm cushion. Flex the foot of your upper leg and place your left hand on your hip to stabilize your pelvis.

↺ Position two

Take a deep breath in and, as you breathe out, draw your navel to your spine and your lats down into your lower back. Your waist lengthens, creating a long, low lift in your upper leg with your hip, knee, and flexed foot facing forward. This is first and foremost a stretch, but the stretch is so strong it turns into a lift. Lower and repeat 10 times on each leg.

INNER THIGHS – BEGINNERS

The muscles of the inner thighs are often completely
forgotten. This exercise will help you to locate and
strengthen them.

⌒ Position one

Sit up against a wall with a straight
back and your legs in a V-shape in
front of you, with your feet flexed, but
don't force this position. Make sure
there is no tension in your shoulders
or neck, and try to press the small of
your back against the wall.
Throughout this exercise keep your
legs straight but not tensed or with
locked knees.

⌒ Position two

Breathe in and, as you breathe out,
move your right leg slowly toward the
left, keeping your foot flexed and
without letting your back come away
from the wall. You should feel the
muscle of your right inner thigh
working. Move your right leg back to its
starting position and move your left leg
toward the right in the same way.
Alternate, 10 times on each leg.

ADDING A WEIGHT

*If you have difficulty feeling this movement in your upper
thigh, place your hand on the inside of your leg and exert a
slight pressure so that you have to work a little harder.*

*As you get stronger, you can use a weight to increase
the effort. Put an ankle weight on the floor just to the
side of your leg, so that the leg has to push it across
the floor. This is actually more effective than
strapping the weight to your leg.*

REMEDIAL LEGS

These exercises were originally developed for specific hip and knee joint problems or injuries in the legs, hence the name. However, they work just as well as ultra-safe strengtheners for the leg muscles.

BEGINNERS

For the best results, do this exercise as slowly and carefully as possible. When your leg is fully extended but still supported, you should feel muscles engaging immediately above your knee.

↻ Position one

Lie back on the floor with your head and shoulders leaning against a firm cushion and most of your spine on the floor. Bend your right leg over a large triangular cushion, and keep your left foot pressed onto the floor.

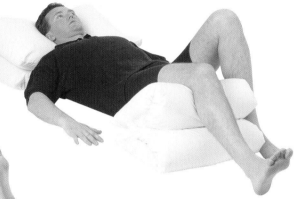

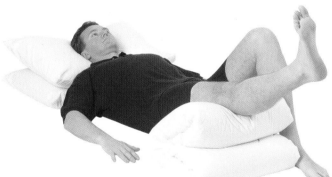

↺ Position two

Breathe in and, as you breathe out, flex your right foot and raise it so that your leg extends out from your knee. Feel as if a piece of string is attached to your big toe and is pulling you up. Don't lift your leg off the cushion but feel it extend fully.

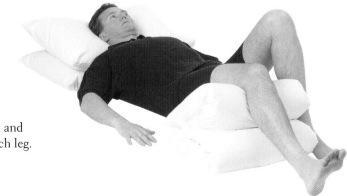

↪ Position three

Return to the starting position and repeat with 10 slow lifts on each leg.

REMEDIAL LEGS – ELEMENTARY

Again, do this exercise slowly, putting as much movement in the foot as you can.

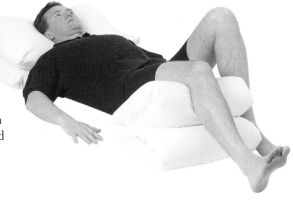

➲ Position one

Lying in exactly the same position as for the previous exercise, extend your right leg as before, with your foot gently flexed.

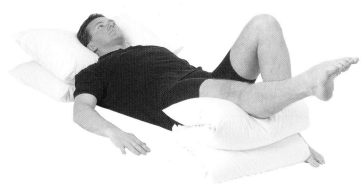

➬ Position two

When your leg is fully extended, point your toe slowly and firmly. Don't let your knee or ankle bend. Your foot should be in one long straight line from your leg. Hold this position for a few seconds.

➲ Position three

Now flex your foot back, feeling the stretch through the back of your knee. Lower your foot to the floor and repeat the sequence 10 times for each leg.

Toning the arms

All of these exercises will strengthen and tone the arm muscles. Later, as the arms become stronger, you can add weights, but for now, concentrate on becoming aware of the muscle groups that you are using.

CHECKLIST

- *Imagine that you are holding a beach ball in front of you so that your arms retain a wide curve throughout.*
- *The movement begins with your hands level with your sternum. Do not allow them to move up to shoulder or chin level, as this can cause tension.*

ARMS – BEGINNERS
➲ **Position one**
Lie on your back with your knees lifted, and your feet flat on the floor a hips' width apart. Check that your spine is not hollowed out or pressed into the floor, and that your neck and shoulders are relaxed. Place your arms in a rounded shape with your hands level with your sternum.

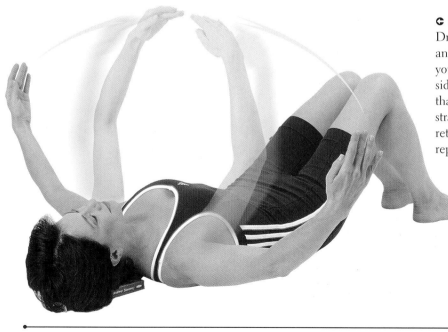

➲ **Position two**
Draw your navel to your spine and, as you breathe in, open your arms straight out to the sides, retaining the curve so that they neither bend nor straighten. Breathe out and return to the starting position, repeating 10 times.

ARMS – ELEMENTARY

This exercise works the triceps, the muscles at the back of the upper arms.

⟳ Position one

Lie on your back with your knees raised and your arms stretched straight up toward the ceiling. Now place your left hand behind your right elbow as a support.

⟲ Position two

Lower your right hand slowly toward your right shoulder, then make a fist and bring it back up in a slow movement into the air. Repeat 10 times and then change arms.

Muscle release

Joseph Pilates' technique uses a series of cushion squeezes.
You will need a cushion that is quite hard so that you have to
exert considerable pressure to squeeze.

CUSHION SQUEEZE
↻ Position one
Lie on your back, with your knees bent
and your feet flat on the floor. Your
arms should be down by your sides,
relaxed. Check that there is no tension
in your shoulders or neck and that the
small of your back is on the floor.
Place the cushion between the thighs.

↻ Position two
Breathe in and, as you breathe out,
draw your navel to your spine, engage
your low buttock muscles, and squeeze
the cushion in a long, slow movement
to the count of ten. Release, and repeat
up to 10 times.

THE CAT

This is a wonderfully sinuous exercise and the aim is to get the movements to flow seamlessly into each other. If you have any back problems, do only positions one and two.

⮑ Position one

Position yourself on your hands and knees – if you can, do this sideways in front of a mirror so that you can check that your back is completely flat, like a tabletop. Your knees should be a hips' width apart so that your shoulders, hips, and knees are aligned.

⮐ Position two

Breathe in and, as you breathe out, draw your navel to your spine, and arch all the way through your back, dropping your head down. Breathe in to return to the starting position.

⮑ Position three

This time as you breathe out, reverse the movement so that your head and your bottom are the highest points, with your back scooped out in a bowl shape. Breathe in and return again to the starting position. Repeat up to 10 times.

Joseph Pilates' Workout: level two

When you feel confident that you can perform all of the exercises in level one correctly and comfortably, without any straining, you are ready to move on to level two.

At this point, the exercises become more complex. You are working several parts of the body simultaneously and so you need to concentrate on using all of the muscle groups properly as you learned at the first level. The key to this is to perform the exercises slowly.

You will also start to use weights. There are two kinds of weights needed: ankle weights and hand weights (dumbbells). The ankle weights are widely available from sports stores and you simply wrap them around your ankle, where indicated in the exercises. If you have dumbbells or you intend to buy them, they should weigh 2 pounds (1 kg). However, you can just as easily use ordinary food cans; hold one in each hand, unless instructed otherwise.

What you have achieved so far

■ *You have started to work at a slow, rhythmic pace and developed deep, even breathing.*

■ *You have isolated the muscles to be used during your program and learned to use them with precision and control.*

■ *Your posture will be improving and you should be losing stored tension.*

Your goals for level two

■ *Build on the exercises of level one to further tone your muscles.*

■ *Work on strengthening key areas, including the use of weights.*

■ *Improve all joint mobility and, in particular, increase suppleness in the back.*

Again, it is important to give yourself plenty of time on this level before going on to the final, advanced program. Do all of the exercises slowly and thoroughly, feeling each group of muscles working at the deepest level.

Some of the exercises from level one are repeated in the program for level two. Begin with the warm-ups (see p. 46-57), then go on to work on the upper body.

Releasing the upper body

In all of these exercises, your navel is held gently against your spine, with your back straight, neck and shoulders relaxed. Always begin the movement by drawing down your lats.

SHOULDER SHRUGS WITH WEIGHTS

This exercise is the same as the one in the warm-up, but now it is done with weights to help you really stretch out your arms and work your lats. You can drop the shoulder shrugs without weights from your warm-up.

<table>
<tr><td>

CHECKLIST

- *Keep your shoulders and neck relaxed as you press back.*
- *If this movement causes you to tense up your neck and shoulders, try it without weights.*
- *Make sure you are breathing deeply and rhythmically to prevent tension.*

</td></tr>
</table>

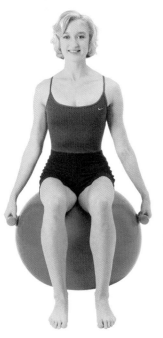

↻ Position three
Relax your shoulders as you breathe out and pull them right down, with the movement coming from your lats, deep into your back. Continue the movement so that you push your arms down and behind you. Feel your upper chest opening up, and you will notice a lift in your sternum. Repeat 10 times.

⌒ Position one
Sit on a chair or support, preferably facing a mirror, with your feet flat on the floor and facing forward. If you have a bolster-type cushion, stand it on its end behind you. Let your arms hang down at your sides, holding a 2-pound (1-kg) weight or can in each hand.

⌒ Position two
Now, breathe in and lift up your shoulders toward your ears. Keep your arms long; don't bend at the elbow.

CLOCK FACE

This is an exercise for the entire lumbar region, rather like a lumbar and sacral massage. The "clock face" does not refer to the circle that your knees are making, but to the circle of the lumbar region.

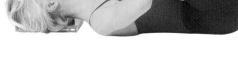

↻ Position one

Lie on your back, with your entire spine stretched out along the floor, your knees drawn up to your chest, and your feet relaxed. Place your hands just below your knees.

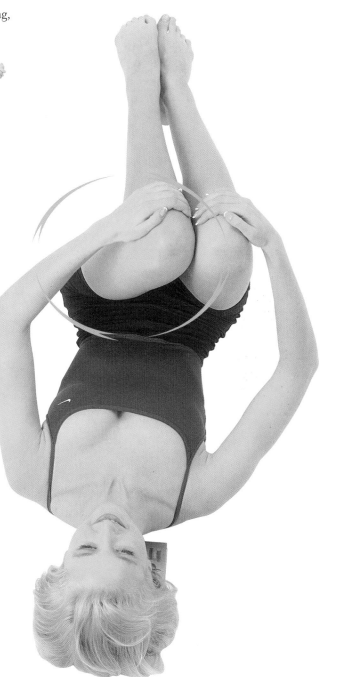

⊃ Position two

Breathe in and, as you breathe out, press your navel back to your spine and keep it there throughout the exercise. Now, with your hands guiding your knees, describe a very small circle with your knees, but concentrate on the larger circle that your back is making on the floor. Don't let your hips tip, and keep the movement deliberately slow and small. Trace 10 circles clockwise, then 10 counterclockwise.

Releasing the upper spine

This is the first of two exercises that are very good for people who tend to store tension in the shoulders, back, or neck. It opens up and loosens this whole area, which, in turn, helps to improve the breathing.

USING THE TOWEL

This exercise uses a rolled-up towel. Take an ordinary hand towel and roll it up tightly, then secure both ends with rubber bands. If the towel feels too uncomfortable, try the exercise without it.

UPPER BACK RELEASE – BEGINNERS
↻ **Position one**
Lie on your back, with your knees raised and your feet flat on the floor. Place a rolled-up towel beneath the middle of your shoulder blades and stretch your arms straight up in the air, fingertips pointing at the ceiling, palms facing forward, but without tension.

↻ **Position two**
Breathe in and, as you breathe out, draw your navel to your spine and take one arm straight back so that your upper arm is next to your ear and, at the same time, take your other arm forward so that it lies against your side, with your fingers pointing down toward your toes. Breathe in again, and, as you breathe out, reverse the position of your arms. Alternate arm movements, breathing deeply, 10 times.

HIP ROLLS – ELEMENTARY

This is a more advanced version of the hip rolls in the warm-up. Here, however, your feet are apart, and this gives you a much greater stretch that you should feel all the way across your body.

➲ Position one

Lie on your back with your feet about 18 inches (45 cm) apart, your neck and spine long and relaxed. Bend your arms and place both hands beneath your head.

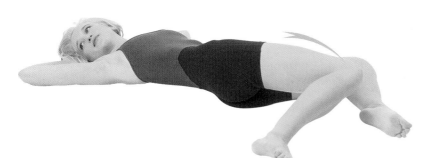

↺ Position two

Breathe in and, as you breathe out, roll your knees toward the floor. If your lower knee can reach the floor easily, try to get the other knee down too. As you stretch, let your head roll in the opposite direction to your knees so that the oblique stretch goes right through your body.

➲ Position three

Breathe in and return to the starting position, then, breathing out, stretch in the opposite direction. Alternate smoothly from side to side, 10 times to each side.

Mobilizing the lower back

Incorrect use of muscles can lead to lower back pain and stiffness. These exercises help release any accumulated tension in this all-important area.

PELVIC TILTS – INTERMEDIATE

This is the third stage of the pelvic tilt, and now arm movements are added to the exercise. However, before you do this, repeat the first two stages (pp. 64-65) as a preparation.

➲ Position one
Breathe out, drawing your navel to your spine, and engage your buttock muscles.

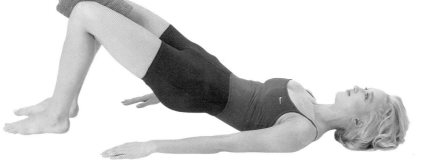

↺ Position two
Start to curl your hips slowly off the floor, keeping your navel drawn toward your spine.

➲ Position three
When your body has curled up as far as it can comfortably go with your abdominals still held in, breathe in and start to raise your arms.

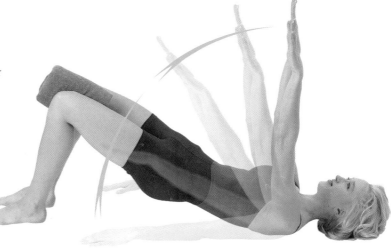

↻ Position four

Holding your body perfectly still, raise your arms above your head, then place them flat on the floor behind you.

↺ Position five

As you breathe out, use your abdominals to curl down vertebra by vertebra, but leave your arms behind you. As you curl down to the floor, you will feel the stretch in your arms increase.

CHECKLIST

- ■ *Make sure you breathe correctly – breathing is a vital part of this exercise.*
- ■ *Try to isolate the vertebrae more each time you repeat the exercise. Ideally, your back should become as sinuous as a snake!*
- ■ *Don't let any tension get into your shoulders, chest, or neck. If they do start to tense, you are coming too far off the floor.*
- ■ *Always begin by pressing down your navel and engaging your low buttock muscles for a moment before you start to move off the floor.*
- ■ *The more slowly you do these pelvic tilts, the more effective they are.*

↺ Position six

Breathe in again and lower your arms to your sides. Repeat 10 times, the slower the better.

Strengthening the central girdle

The following exercises are the next steps in the series that began with the buttock squeeze (see p. 68), which you should repeat 10 times before going on to the next ones.

HEEL LIFTS
After you have completed the buttock squeeze, remove the cushion from between your thighs for this exercise.

↻ Position one
Lie in the same position as for the buttock squeeze. Breathe in deeply and, as you breathe out, draw your navel to your spine, and engage the muscles at the base of your buttocks so that all these muscles are working. Hold this position throughout the exercise.

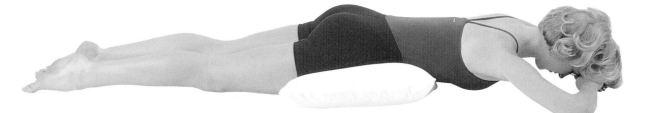

↻ Position two
Holding the position, breathe in and, as you breathe out, slowly bend your right leg from your knee directing your heel toward your buttocks. Breathe in and lower your foot slowly, feeling the stretch in your hamstring, still holding your abdominal muscles.

Relax, take a deep breath in, and then breathe out to draw your navel to your spine, as before. Repeat the heel lifts 10 times on the other leg.

PREPARATION FOR THE ARROW

The arrow is one of the most in-depth exercises for the whole central girdle. It is presented in full on p. 110 in level three, and this introductory exercise strengthens the muscles that will be used.

↻ Position one
Lie in the same position as for the previous exercise, but this time with your arms stretched out above your head.

↻ Position two
Breathe in, breathe out, draw your navel to your spine, and engage your buttock muscles. Draw down your lats and trapezius muscles so that your arms are drawn down and your head lifts up slightly, in line with your spine. Lower and repeat, working up to 10 repetitions.

↻ Position three
Spend a few moments in the rest position (see p. 69).

CHECKLIST

- *Don't try to lift your upper body far from the floor; this is essentially a long, low stretch.*
- *Make sure your abdominal and buttock muscles are engaged throughout. Rest if you feel tired.*

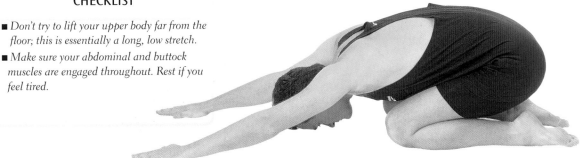

Toning the legs

Your legs should now be feeling stronger and you should be much more aware of their various muscles groups. The exercises on the next four pages work on toning, strengthening, and stretching the legs further.

SIDE LIFTS
In this exercise, the leg lifts further than in the exercise on p. 70. Keep checking that your knee, foot, and hips are all parallel and facing forward.

↺ Position one
Lie on your side, with your back flat against the wall, your hips parallel and facing forward, and with a small cushion to support your waist. Place a cushion or towel between your head and your lower, outstretched arm. Place your other hand on the floor for support.

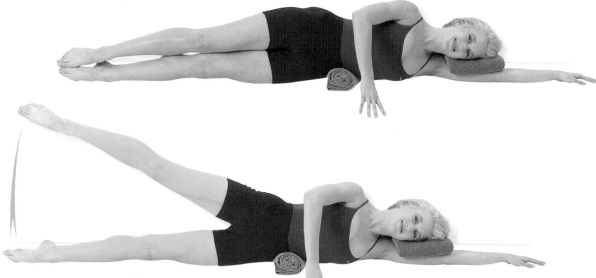

↻ Position two
Breathe in and, as you breathe out, draw your navel to your spine and raise your top leg with your knee facing forward. You should be able to feel the muscle working all the way up your thigh. Lower and repeat 10 times on each leg.

↺ Position three
When you can raise one leg with ease, you can do a double leg lift. Keep the lift low (it is a much harder exercise to do) and stop if you feel a strain. Work slowly up to 10 repetitions.

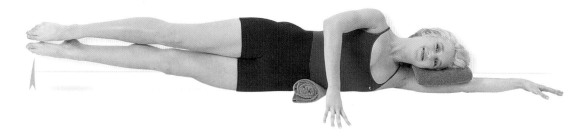

INNER THIGHS – ELEMENTARY

This exercise and the following one strengthen the muscles of the inner thigh that are often forgotten. You are using the same muscles as in the exercise on p. 71. If you have difficulty isolating the correct muscles, repeat the earlier exercise.

↻ Position one

Lie on your side, with your back flat against a wall. Make sure your hips and shoulders are in line and keep them next to the wall throughout the exercise, even when your legs are moving. Put a big cushion or rolled-up towel in front of you and rest your top knee on it. Rest your head on your arm and stretch your lower leg away from you.

↻ Position two

Breathe in and, as you breathe out, press your navel back toward the wall. With your foot gently pointed, extend your lower leg. Keeping your knee facing squarely forward, lift your heel slowly. Breathe in as you lower it, and try to make the whole movement smooth. Repeat for 10 lifts each side.

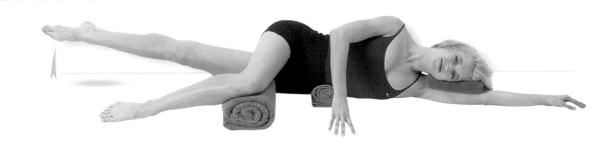

FEELING STRONGER?

This exercise repeats the movements of the previous one, but this time with the addition of ankle weights. Don't go on to this until you can do the exercise effortlessly without using weights.

OUTER THIGHS – ELEMENTARY

This exercise repeats the one in level one but now you use an ankle weight.

⏻ Position one

Strap on ankle weights and lie on your side with your back flat against a wall. Let your lower arm stretch out and place a pillow folded double between this arm and your head, with another to support your waist. Bend your lower leg and place your upper leg on a large, firm cushion. Flex the foot of your upper leg and place your upper arm flat against the wall.

CHECKLIST

- *Keep your back completely flat against the wall, with your hips facing directly forward.*
- *Keep your legs parallel.*
- *The slower the movement and more stretched out your leg, the better it is.*

⏻ Position two

Take a deep breath in and, as you breathe out, draw your navel to your spine and your lats down into your lower back. Let your upper arm stretch out against the wall so that your waist lengthens, creating a long, low lift in your upper leg with your hip, knee, and flexed foot facing forward. Lower and repeat 10 times on each leg.

GLUTEAL STRETCHES

There are two stages of this stretch for the gluteal muscles of the buttocks, the first one being easier. It is also a diagonal stretch for the back.

BE GENTLE

- *Don't force the turn. If you feel any strain in the back, stop immediately.*
- *Make sure that the hand on your right leg is on the thigh, not the knee.*

STAGE ONE
↻ Position one

Sit on the floor with your legs straight, and your right hand supporting you. Cross your right leg over your left with your knee raised, and your right foot behind your left knee.

↺ Position two

Turn smoothly to the right. Feel the stretch starting in your buttocks, and going through your upper body until your head turns. Hold the stretch, return to the starting position, and repeat four times on each side.

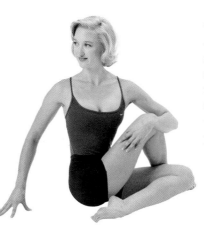

STAGE TWO
↻ Position one

Sit up, and bend your left leg, bringing your foot toward your buttock. Cross your right leg over your left, placing your left hand on your raised thigh.

↻ Position two

As before, turn toward your supporting hand in a slow, smooth, controlled movement, feeling the stretch move gradually through your body. Keep your back upright.

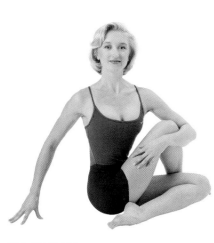

Strengthening the abdominals

The abdominal muscles are central to balance, strength, and posture, but that strength can take some time to acquire. Do these exercises very gently and stop if you see the abdominals start to bulge out. This means you are putting too much strain both on the abdominal muscles and those in the back, and you are probably trying to take the movement further than is safe as yet. The oblique abdominals are the muscles you feel when you twist or bend.

SIT-UPS

Only go onto these sit-ups when you can do those in level one with ease. Nothing is accomplished by straining to come up a long way; it just makes your abdominal muscles bulge out and puts a strain on your back. It's better to keep the movement smaller and more controlled.

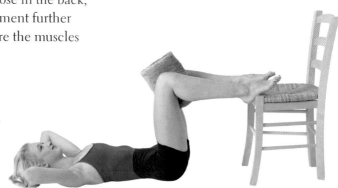

⌒ Position one
Lie on your back with your feet on a chair so that your knees form a right angle. Place a bolster or cushion between your knees. Place your hands behind your head and check that your shoulders and neck are relaxed.

⟳ Position two
Breathe in and, as you breathe out, draw your navel to your spine and lift your head and shoulders off the floor, keeping your chin dropped and your shoulders and neck relaxed. Don't struggle to sit all the way up. It's much more important that your abdominals are still in a scooped-in shape; if they start to bulge out or quiver, you have come up too far. Return slowly, rolling down to the starting position. Repeat the exercise 10 times.

OBLIQUE SIT-UPS

The oblique abdominals are likely to be under-developed compared to the central ones, so don't attempt to come too far off the floor at first.

➲ Position one

Lie on your back with your knees raised. Place your left hand behind your head and the right on top of your abdomen, so you can feel whether your abdominal muscles are working properly.

↻ Position two

Breathe in and, as you breathe out, draw your navel to your spine and your lats down your back. Now roll over toward the right as if you were getting out of bed. Stretch out your right hand so that the oblique muscles work against it. When your oblique abdominal muscles are really strong, the aim is to get all your lats off the floor – but very few people manage this! Come up only as far as your abdominal muscles can hold without bulging or quivering. Lower and change sides, working up to 10 repeats on each side.

SINGLE LEG STRETCHES

This (and the double leg stretch, see p. 120) are two of the best-known of the original exercises Pilates devised. The names are somewhat misleading as they both entail a great deal more work than a simple stretch of the leg!

CHECKLIST

■ *Hold your basic position – navel to spine and head and shoulders curled up – throughout the exercise. Don't lie down fully until you have finished.*

■ *Try to maintain a small turnout from the hips all the way through; you will be more aware of this as you stretch your leg away.*

➲ Position one

Lie on your back and draw your knees to your chest. Keep your knees a shoulders' width apart, with your feet touching. Draw your navel to your spine and curve your upper torso forward as you slide your hands down to your ankles.

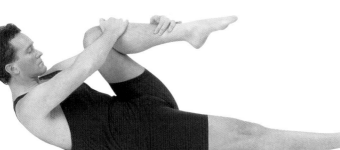

↺ Position two

Breathe in and, as you breathe out, stretch out your right leg and draw your left knee to your chest, keeping your left hand on your left ankle. This helps to keep your ankle in line with your knee.

➲ Position three

Breathe in, then breathe out as you stretch. Change legs so that this time the left is stretched away from you. Repeat, alternating, 10 times on each leg.

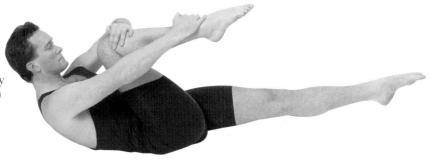

Strengthening the arms

These exercises will strengthen and tone the arm muscles.
Practice first without weights, then, as your arms become
stronger, you can add the weights. You can use dumbbells up
to 2 pounds (1 kg) or simply hold food cans in your hands.

CHECKLIST

- *Hold your arms in a wide curve throughout.*
- *Always start with your hands level with your sternum; avoid the tendency to hold them much higher up toward shoulder level.*

ARM WEIGHTS – BEGINNERS

This exercise was done in level one without
weights. If your arms still find this a strain,
continue as before.

ↄ Position one

Lie on your back with your knees lifted, feet
flat on the floor and a hips' width apart.
Check that the small of your back is pressed
against the floor and your neck and
shoulders are relaxed. Let your arms form a
rounded shape with your hands level with
your sternum. If you are using weights, hold
one in each hand.

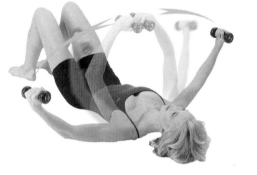

↻ Position two

Breathe in, draw your navel
to your spine, and open your
arms straight out to the
sides, retaining their curved
shape. Breathe out and
return to the starting
position. Repeat 10 times.

ARM WEIGHTS – ELEMENTARY

This is a new exercise, so try it without
weights to start with and be sure that you
keep the arms curved throughout.

ↄ Position one

Lie on your back, as in the previous
exercise, with your arms in a long
oval shape. If you are not using a
weight, clasp your fingers loosely
together. If you have a weight, hold
it in both hands.

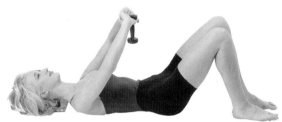

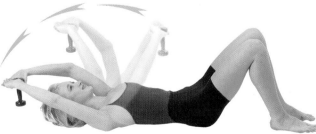

↺ Position two

Breathe out to draw your navel to your
spine and take your hands back behind
your head, keeping your arms in an oval.
Don't go too far or your abdominals will
bulge out. Breathe out and return to the
starting position, and repeat 10 times.

Strengthening the back

This exercise is for the muscles of the back, often neglected or completely forgotten. You need to do this exercise very slowly, focusing all of your attention on your back so that you become fully aware of these muscles.

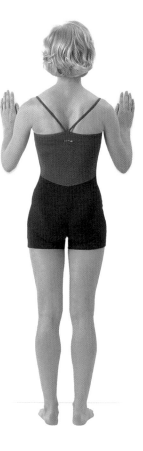

↪ **Position one**
Face a wall, with your toes almost touching it. Your feet should be a hips' width apart. Be sure your back is straight and there is no tension in your neck and shoulders. Place your palms flat on the wall at shoulder height.

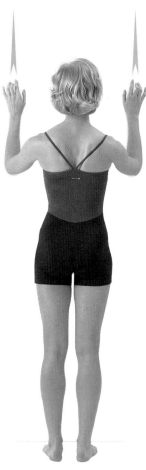

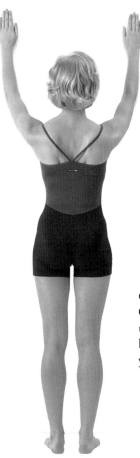

↷ **Position two**
Start to crawl your fingers very slowly up the wall. As your hands move gradually upward, feel the separate muscles that are being used in your back.

↺ **Position three**
Continue the crawling movement until your arms are outstretched but without tension. Do not lift your shoulders to get higher.

➲ Position four

In a long, sweeping movement, slowly take your arms down. You should be describing as large a circle as you can without allowing tension to creep in. Check that your neck and shoulders are relaxed, replace your hands on the wall, and repeat two or three times.

LOCATING THE BACK MUSCLES

Because the back muscles are so underused, people often don't even realize that they are there! This exercise locates and strengthens them, and teaches you how to move your arms without creating tension in your back, neck, and shoulders.

Working the legs

REMEDIAL LEGS – INTERMEDIATE

This is the third stage of the remedial leg exercises and now includes a turnout. Remember, turnout always originates in the hip socket, not the leg or foot. Before you do this exercise, repeat the first two in the series (pp. 72–73).

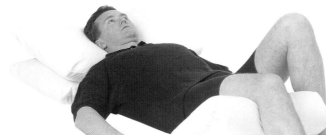

↻ Position one
Lie on your back with your right knee supported on the cushion, as in the previous exercises in the series. Breathe in and, as you breathe out, lift your lower leg and extend it so that it is still on the cushion but the muscles above your knee are engaged and your entire leg is stretched out.

↪ Position two
When your leg is fully extended, turn it out from your hip, not your foot, then rotate it back to a parallel position and lower it. Repeat 10 times slowly on each leg.

QUAD STRETCH

You will feel this exercise as a strong stretch all the way up the front of your thigh. You need to find a strong, high surface such as a table or a kitchen counter to take your weight.

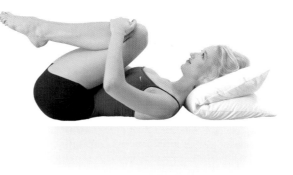

➲ Position one

Sit on the very edge of the table, then lie down with a cushion to support your head and neck, with your knees drawn gently up to your chest.

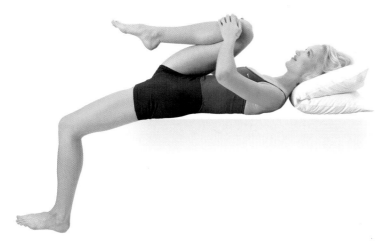

↻ Position two

Breathe in and, as you breathe out, draw your navel to your spine and make sure your entire back is in contact with the table. Let your left leg hang down over the edge of the table, while you hold your right gently to the chest, keeping your abdominals engaged and your entire back on the table. Hold the position for at least three minutes. The weight of your overhanging leg will open up your hip socket.

➲ Position three

Keeping your abdominal muscles firmly engaged and your back in contact with the table, breathe in and bring your left leg back to the center. Now, breathing out, let your right leg hang down over the edge. Repeat 10 times with alternate legs.

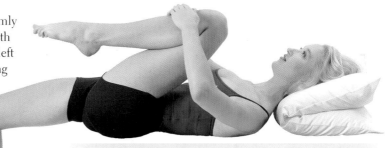

HAMSTRING STRETCH

The hamstring muscles are often very tight, particularly in women who wear high-heeled shoes. Do not force the stretch; just take it as far as you need to in order to feel a stretch, but not a strain.

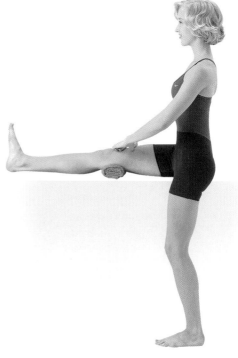

➲ Position one

Sit on the edge of a bed, with one leg straight out in front of you and the other foot on the floor, making sure your hips are square. Place a small cushion underneath the knee of your stretched leg and flex your foot. Make sure that you are sitting up straight with your navel pulling back toward your spine.

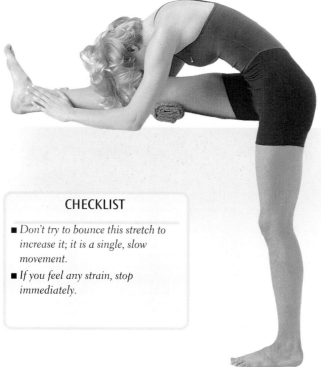

CHECKLIST

■ *Don't try to bounce this stretch to increase it; it is a single, slow movement.*

■ *If you feel any strain, stop immediately.*

↩ Position two

Breathe in and, as you breathe out, lean your upper body forward smoothly, keeping your foot flexed. You will feel the stretch in the back of your leg, in the hamstring. When you reach the limit of your stretch, hold it for a few seconds. This is a slow, gentle stretch, so do not reach forward too far. Breathe in and return to the starting position. Repeat 10 times on each side.

CUSHION SQUEEZE – ELEMENTARY

This cushion squeeze is much harder than the one in level one, and you will feel it very strongly in the inner thigh muscles. Do the cushion squeeze on p. 76 as a warm-up for this one.

RELAX

■ *Because this exercise requires a lot of effort, it is very easy for tension to creep in. Between each squeeze, check your neck, arms, back, shoulders, and even your face. Relax and repeat.*

↻ Position one

Lie with your back completely flat on the floor, and your legs straight and stretched out in front of you. Place a firm cushion between your feet, which should be gently flexed.

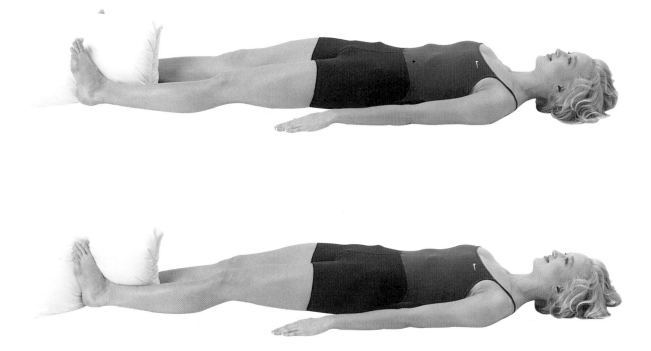

↻ Position two

Breathe in and, as you breathe out, draw your navel to your spine and engage your low buttock muscles. Now squeeze the cushion between your feet. You should feel the entire length of your inner thigh muscles working. Release, and repeat 10 times.

Joseph Pilates' Workout: level three

When you can perform all of the exercises of levels one and two with ease, you are ready to go on to the final stage of Pilates' exercises in level three.

Don't feel you have to rush into doing this. It is much better to spend more time strengthening the muscles than to attempt to do exercises that your body isn't quite ready for, and so won't be able to do correctly. All of the central girdle – lats, abdominals, buttocks – need to be very strong for some of these exercises, especially those like the advanced sit-ups, the Arrow, the Dog, or the double leg stretches.

It is still very important to prepare the body before such exercises, so always do the warm-up first and spend time on these deceptively simple exercises; they are the foundation for all of the more difficult ones.

What you have achieved

- *You will by now have seen a very noticeable improvement in your muscle tone and strength.*

- *Your posture will be more centered and graceful, and your limbs will be moving with less effort and more precision.*

- *You will have increased mobility and suppleness.*

Your goals for level three and beyond

- *Further muscular strengthening and toning, particularly of the central girdle.*

- *Improved coordination in more complex exercises.*

- *A sense of posture and placement that becomes natural poise in all daily movements.*

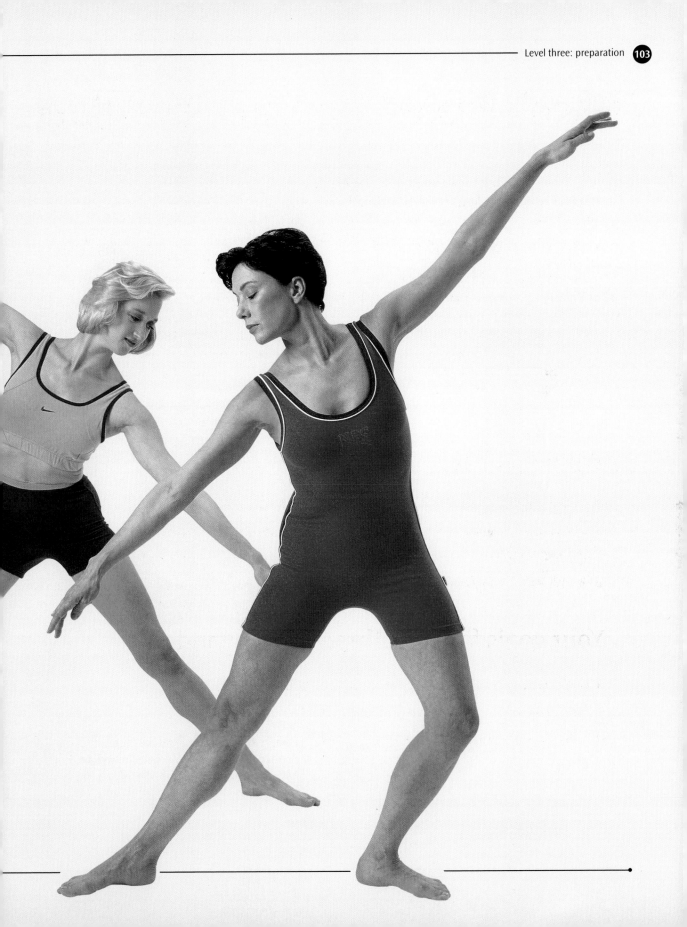

Releasing the spine

This exercise will be a good release for you if you have a tendency to store tension in the shoulders, back, or neck. It follows on from the first upper back release (p. 62), opens up the whole area, and improves the breathing.

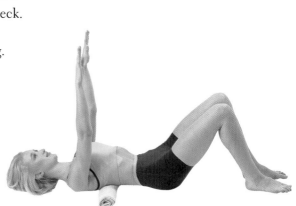

UPPER BACK RELEASE – ELEMENTARY
➲ Position one
Lie on your back with your knees raised and a rolled-up towel supporting your upper back. In this exercise, the arms describe an entire circle. Begin with your arms raised, and your fingers pointing up to the ceiling.

↺ Position two
Breathe in and, as you breathe out, press your navel to your spine and take one arm back behind your head and one forward on the floor, with your fingers pointing to your toes.

➲ Position three
Rotate your arms out to the sides, simultaneously, until they are both at 90° to the body. Now turn your palms over and continue the circle until your arms have changed positions.

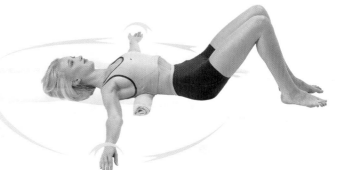

↺ Position four
Bring both arms back up to the starting position, pointing straight up to the ceiling, then begin again with your other arm going back first. Alternate for 10 repetitions.

UPPER BACK RELEASE – INTERMEDIATE

This exercise extends the arm and back movements used in the earlier versions on pp. 60-61. As before, make sure you are using your back muscles rather than your shoulders.

➲ Position two
With your upper arms staying close to your sides, begin to open your chest by turning your hands slowly outward.

➲ Position one
Sit on a chair, with your knees bent at right angles, and your shoulders even and relaxed. Bend your arms at the elbows, keeping the upper arms close to your sides and your palms facing down.

➲ Position three
Now let your upper arms open up too as your hands move further behind you. Don't lift your shoulders.

➲ Position five
To release your back, wrap your arms around your chest, drop your head, and draw your navel to your spine as you breathe out. Repeat 10 times.

➲ Position four
Extend your arms behind you as far as they will go without distorting or lifting your shoulders. Feel the squeeze in your back as your shoulder blades push together.

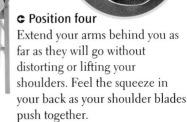

Mobilizing the spine

This is the final stage of the pelvic tilts and, as its name implies, the most advanced. It is a difficult movement and not one that should be tried until your abdominals are strong. As with the previous exercises, begin with a deep breath and, as you breathe out, draw your navel to your spine, tighten your buttock muscles, and curl your spine off the floor in a smooth curve. Begin with some of the more basic pelvic tilts (see pp. 64-65 and 84-85) as a warm-up.

> ### IMPORTANT
>
> *This strenuous exercise is particularly tough on the abdominal muscles. Do each position properly rather than immediately going through the sequence 10 times. If you feel any pain in your back, or if your stomach starts to bulge out or quiver, stop at once.*

PELVIC TILTS – ADVANCED
➲ Position one
Lie on your back with your knees raised and your arms, neck, and back relaxed. Put a cushion between your thighs.

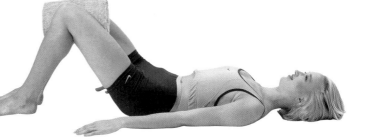

↻ Position two
Take a deep breath, then, as you breathe out, draw your navel down toward your spine, feeling it flatten out along the floor. Squeeze the muscles at the very base of your buttocks, but try to avoid squeezing the hamstrings in your thighs. Let the squeeze draw your body up, tightening your inner thighs and raising your body, vertebra by vertebra, in an arc from the floor.

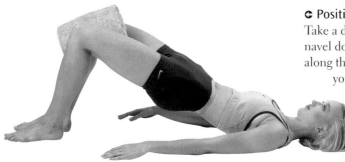

➲ Position three
When your body has curled up as far as it can comfortably go with your abdominals still held in, breathe in and lift your arms up above your head and put them flat on the floor behind you.

↻ Position four

As you breathe out, curl down vertebra by vertebra, but leaving your arms behind you. As your spine curls down to the floor, you will feel the stretch in your arms increase.

↻ Position five

Breathe out, place your hands very gently beneath your head, and raise your upper body very slightly off the floor, with your nose pointing straight up to the ceiling.

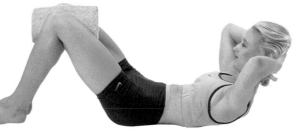

↻ Position six

Now, continue to rise up, so your head faces forward and you feel the curve reach the middle of your ribs.

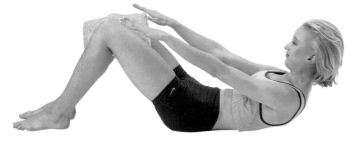

↻ Position seven

Finally, release your hands from behind your head and stretch them toward your thighs, so that the movement is felt in your lower abdominal muscles. Build up to 10 repetitions, resting when necessary.

The girdle of strength

The following exercises extend the work of the heel lifts in level two, making the lifts harder each time. However, add weights or the rolled-up towel only when you are completely comfortable with the basic exercise and, if you feel you are taking the strain in your back, remove the weights at once.

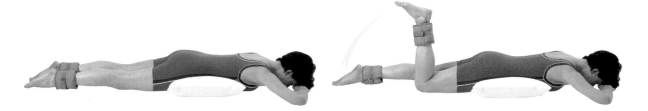

HEEL LIFTS WITH WEIGHTS
∩ Position one
Strap on ankle weights and lie on your front with a pillow beneath your abdomen and your face resting on your hands. Breathe in deeply and, as you breathe out, draw your navel to your spine and engage the muscles at the base of your buttocks so that all these muscles are working. Remember to hold this position throughout the exercise.

∩ Position two
Holding the position, breathe in and, as you breathe out, slowly bend your lower leg from the knee as far as it will go in the direction of your buttocks. Make sure that the heel does not move from the center line. Breathe in and lower your foot, still holding the position. Repeat 10 times for each leg.

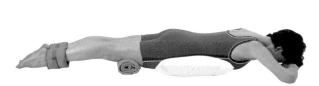

HEEL LIFTS WITH TOWEL
∩ Position one
Do this exercise first without weights, but avoid it if you have a knee injury or feel any strain. Lie face down with a pillow under your abdomen. Place a rolled-up towel under your legs, just above the knee. Rest your face on your hands and keep your upper body relaxed.

∩ Position two
Breathe in and, as you breathe out, draw your navel to your spine, engage your low buttock muscles, and hold this position throughout the exercise. Slowly bend your lower leg from the knee, following the instructions from the previous exercise. Lower and repeat 10 times, then repeat 10 times on the other leg.

STOMACH STRETCHES

For this exercise to work properly, you need to keep your navel pulled well into your spine throughout. Start with just one or two repetitions, building up to five as you feel stronger.

↻ Position one

Lie face down, with your arms and legs stretched out, hands and feet a hips' width apart, palms down, and legs turned out with your feet pointed. Use a pillow under your stomach and hips to support your lower back. Breathe in and, as you breathe out, pull your navel up to your spine and feel a gap open up between you and the floor. Hold this position throughout the exercise.

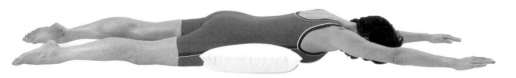

➔ Position two

Breathe in and, as you breathe out, keep the stretch in your arms and legs, and lift your left arm and right leg approximately 2 inches (5 cm) off the floor.

↻ Position three

Breathe in to lower. Breathe out and repeat with your right arm and left leg.

➔ Position four

Breathe in and, breathing out, lift both arms and legs 2 inches (5 cm) off the floor. Repeat the whole sequence five times.

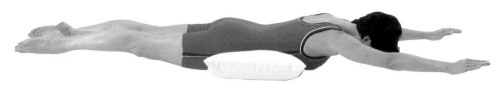

THE ARROW

The Arrow uses every area of the central girdle; the lats, the abdominal muscles, and the buttocks all work in unison. Always start with the buttock squeezes and the heel lifts (pp. 68-69 and 86-87) before you practice the Arrow so you can check that all your muscles are working to their maximum before you start!

↻ Position one
Lie face down on a hard bed or on the floor with a cushion beneath your abdomen. Place a pillow beneath your forehead so that you can look down comfortably. Put your arms by your sides, with your fingers pointing to your feet.

↻ Position two
Breathe in and, as you breathe out, draw your navel to your spine and squeeze your low buttock muscles together. Lift your arms toward the ceiling, pull your shoulder blades down toward your pelvis, and lift your sternum and head away from the floor.

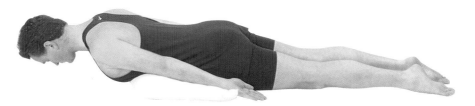

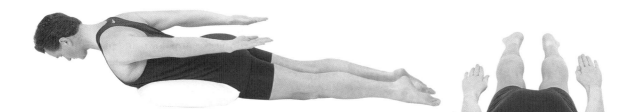

↻↻ Position three
Neither your arms nor your upper body should come high off the floor; this is a long stretch rather than a lift. Breathe in and come down, and repeat 10 times.

REST POSITION WITH HELP

After the Arrow, take a short rest. This rest position is an extension of the one in level one. If you are working with a partner, you could ask for help with this stretch. Ask your partner to place one hand at each end of your spine, and pull the hands gently further apart.

CHECKLIST FOR THE ARROW

- *Don't try to come up too far from the floor. This is really a long two-way stretch.*
- *Keep your palms facing the ceiling.*
- *Don't let your neck or shoulders tense.*
- *Keep your arms straight, but not stiff.*
- *Breathe very slowly and deeply.*

➲ **Position one**
From the Arrow position draw your body back so that you are sitting back on your heels, with your arms stretched out in front of you.

↻ **Position two**
Bring one arm down and place it next to your side, with your fingers pointing to your toes. Then bring your second arm down to your side. You may find it more comfortable to let your head roll to one side. Stay like this for a few moments and relax.

Releasing the back

In this third stage of the hip rolls, we show the exercise with arms outstretched; however, you may find it helpful at first to hold onto a heavy piece of furniture. Position it behind you so you can hold on with your arms behind your head. The legs of a heavy chair or table, about 2 to 3 feet (60-90 cm) apart, would be ideal.

HIP ROLLS – INTERMEDIATE
➲ Position one

Lie on your back with your arms extended out to the sides or holding onto the furniture to steady yourself. Make a right angle with your knees so that your thighs are vertical and your calves are parallel to the floor.

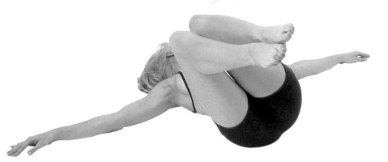

↻ Position two

Breathe in and, as you breathe out, keeping your knees together, stretch them slowly to one side, feeling an oblique stretch across your body. The movement should start in the top buttock for maximum stretch.

➲ Position three

You will have to let your hips come off the floor, but your shoulders should stay down. Your head should turn in the opposite direction from your legs each time. Alternate for 10 slow rolls each side.

HIP ROLLS – ADVANCED

When you can do the previous exercise comfortably, try this exercise. It requires even more strength in your abdominals as they have to sustain the weight of your whole leg.

↻ Position one

Lie on your back as in the previous exercise, using a piece of furniture to anchor you if you wish, or with your arms stretched out to the sides. Your legs should be stretched out on the floor.

➲ Position two

As you breathe in, bend your left knee slowly and draw it up toward your chest, keeping your foot pointed. Keep your right leg stretched out on the floor.

↻ Position three

Roll your left leg over, still bent, across the right. Turn your head to face the opposite direction.

➲ Position four

Stretch your leg, flex your foot, and let the weight of your leg help drop it toward the floor. Leave it there for a moment, feeling the stretch. Point your foot. Breathe in, bend your leg, and use your stomach muscles to roll back and bring your knee back to your chest. Breathe out and slowly straighten your leg back to the starting position. Change legs and repeat the exercise on the other side. Alternate, 10 times.

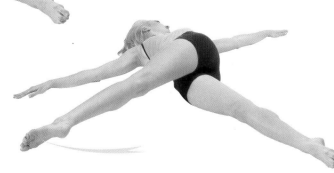

SIDE TWISTS

This exercise combines a side stretch with a twist. It opens up the sides and works on the waist – but you must be careful to keep your hips completely still while you are doing it.

➲ Position one

Sit up straight, with your legs stretched out in front of you. Bend your left leg so that your foot is level with your right knee, and allow your left knee to drop toward the floor.

➲ Position two

Stretch out your spine, keeping your neck and head in alignment, and raise your arms above your head, with your fingers pointing to the ceiling. Breathe in. As you breathe out, move your torso smoothly around to face your bent knee, keeping your hips parallel.

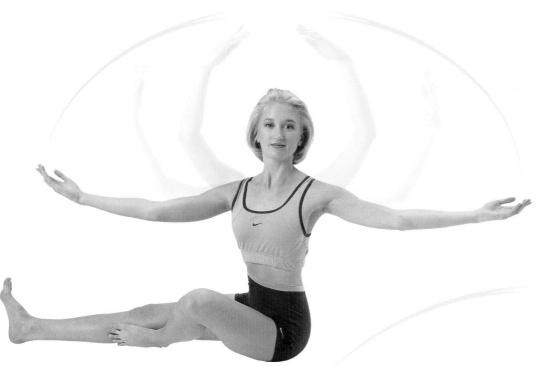

⌒ Position three

Lower your arms straight out to the sides. Your palms should be facing the ceiling, and your hips should not have moved. Check that your shoulders are relaxed, and your back and chest are open.

⤺ Position four

Breathe out and curve your body smoothly down toward the straight leg, bringing your upper arm in a long overhead curve, with your lower leg reaching toward the inside of your foot. Hold the stretch for a few moments, if you can.

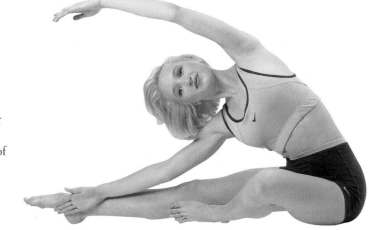

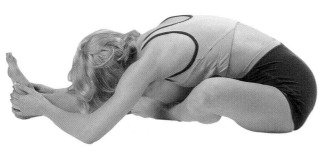

⤼ Position five

Breathe in, turn parallel, and stretch out along your leg. Return to the starting position and repeat four times on each side.

Toning the legs

The first exercise is a repeat of previous ones, but is now made harder by using ankle weights. Keep checking that your knee, foot, and hips are all parallel and facing forward for the full benefit from this exercise. The second exercise, Rondes de Jambes, is based on ballet barre work but, because you are lying down, it ensures that you stay in alignment, which can often get distorted if you are standing at the barre. It demands a great deal of strength in the abdominals, as well as in the legs.

OUTER THIGHS – INTERMEDIATE
↻ Position one

Strap on your ankle weights. Lie on your side, with your back flat against the wall, your hips parallel and facing forward, and with a small cushion to support your waist. Place your hand just below your hip and gently press down toward the floor. This will ensure that the work is concentrated on the outer thigh.

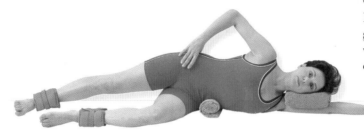

↻ Position two

Breathe in and, as you breathe out, draw your navel to your spine and raise your top leg with a gently flexed foot, and your knee facing forward. You should be able to feel the muscle working all the way up your thigh.

↻ Position three

Raise your leg to its full extent, checking with your hand that your hip stays parallel and doesn't shift. Lower, and repeat 10 times on each leg.

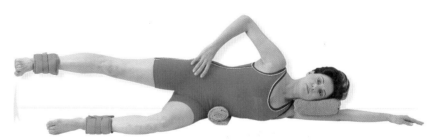

RONDES DE JAMBES

Literally, this means "leg circles," but the circle is very small, traced with the toe.

↷ Position one

Lie on your side, with your back flat against the wall, your hips parallel, with a cushion under your waist, and your top hand on your hip. Bend your top leg. Stretch your lower arm out and rest your head on it.

↻ Position two

As you breathe out, raise your lower leg. It will not be able to come very far off the ground.

↻ Position three

Now, rotate from your hip so your leg is turned out, and point your foot.

Describe four circles with your toe, clockwise and counterclockwise. Repeat 10 times with each leg.

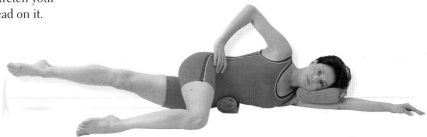

Strengthening the abdominals

When you can do the sit-ups from level two with ease, you can make it harder by changing your position so that your feet are on the floor, with your knees raised, instead of resting on a chair. This way, you have further to go!

➲ Position one

Lie on your back with your knees raised and your feet flat on the floor. Put your hands behind your head. Check that your shoulders and neck are relaxed.

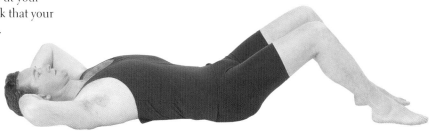

➲ Position two

Breathe in and, as you breathe out, draw your navel to your spine and lift your head and shoulders off the floor, keeping your chin dropped and your neck and shoulders relaxed.

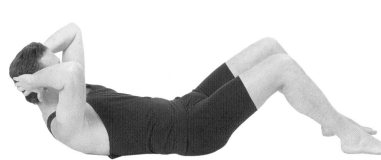

➲ Position three

Stretch your arms toward your knees. As always, don't struggle to sit all the way up. It's much more important that your abdominals are still in a scooped-in shape; if they start to bulge out or quiver, you have come up too far.

When you have come up as far as you can, extend your arms in front of you. This will raise your body slightly further. Return slowly, rolling down to the starting position, and repeat 10 times.

THE OBLIQUE STRENGTHENER

This exercise works the oblique abdominal muscles and trims the waist. Begin with positions one and two and go on to position three only when you can do the first part comfortably.

↻ Position one

Lie on the floor with your knees bent, your spine straight, and your navel pressing lightly toward your spine. Put your right arm straight on the floor by your side, and your left bent at the elbow, with your hand lightly holding your head.

STABILIZER

To help you hold this position easily and to keep your knees in place, put a cushion between your knees as a stabilizer. You could also tuck your feet under a piece of furniture, or ask a friend to hold them in place.

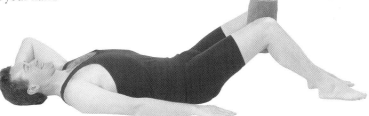

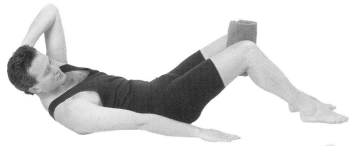

↻ Position two

Breathe in and, as you breathe out, reach your right arm toward your right thigh, and roll your head and neck up from the floor, without straining or tensing your shoulders. As you come off the floor, turn so that your left elbow and shoulder lift toward your right knee.

↻ Position three

Holding your body in place with your abdominal muscles, raise your right arm.

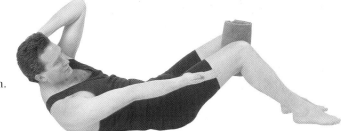

↻ Position four

Now raise your left arm. Turn the palm of your right hand up and bring your left arm across your body, placing your left palm over your right. Stretch both arms beyond your left knee. Place your right hand behind your head, keeping the left palm face down. Return to position one.

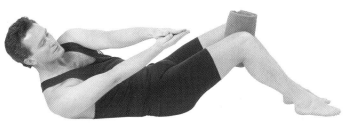

DOUBLE LEG STRETCH

Before doing the double leg stretch, it is a good idea to do 10 single leg stretches from p. 94 (on each leg) as a warm-up. This is a strenuous exercise, so don't expect to be able to do 10 repetitions to start with; just do 3 or 4 well, and work up gradually.

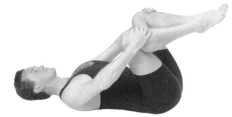

↺ Position one

Lie on the floor with your back flat, and your knees bent up toward your chest, a shoulders' width apart. Place your hands just below your knees and check that your neck and shoulders are relaxed.

➲ Position two

Breathe in and, as you breathe out, draw your navel to your spine, keeping your tailbone on the floor, and curl your head and shoulders up off the floor, with your chin down toward, but not on, your chest.

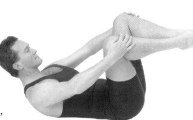

↻ Position three

Breathe in and stretch out your arms and legs together so that they are at a 60° angle to the floor. Turn out your legs, squeezing your inner thighs together.

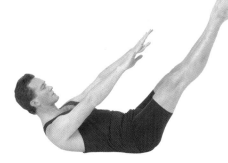

↻ Position five

As you breathe in, continue the circle of your arms out to the sides and then up toward 60° again. Point your toes.

Breathe out, slowly bending both knees and elbows, placing your hands just below your knees and resting your head and upper back on the floor. Repeat the whole sequence up to 10 times.

↺ Position four

Keeping your legs and feet where they are, breathe out and stretch your arms up to the ceiling, then back behind your head, brushing past your ears. Turn your palms out.

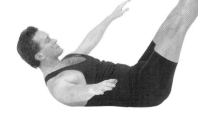

THE DOG

This exercise has some similarities to the Cat (see p. 77) – but it requires a lot more strength and a good sense of balance.

➲ Position one

Begin in the same position as the Cat, with the weight evenly distributed between your hands and knees, your feet a hips' width apart, and your back flat as a tabletop all the way through to the top of your head.

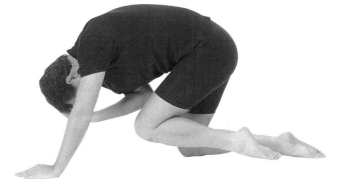

➲ Position two

Breathe in, and gently arch your back as you curl your right elbow and left knee under your torso. You are now balancing on your left hand and right leg.

↻ Position three

Now, breathe out and extend your right arm and left leg and stretch them out fully, keeping them parallel with the floor.

Repeat the exercise at least 5 times, then change arms and legs, and repeat 5 times on the other side.

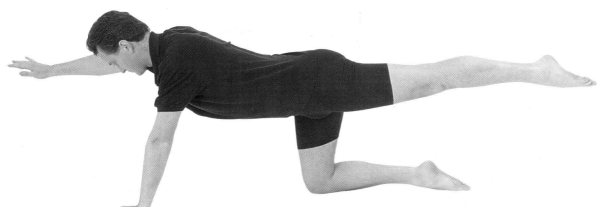

Releasing the upper body

Begin with the four upper body exercises to center yourself and to release tension in your neck, back, or shoulders. Start with the shoulder shrug with weights (p. 80), then the two openings (pp. 60-61 and 105), and then the Cossack (p. 63).

ARMS AND LATS

The following exercise builds on the upper body work and stretches out the lats even more. For this exercise, you will need a short pole (about 2 to 3 feet [60-90 cm] long) or a rolled-up towel, secured with rubber bands.

➲ Position one

Lie on your back with your knees raised. Check your alignment – you should be in a long, straight line from the base of your spine to the nape of your neck. Hold the pole or towel in your hands, which should be about 18 inches (45 cm) apart.

↻ Position two

Breathe in and, as you breathe out, draw your navel to your spine and draw your hands toward your face, bending your arms at the elbows. Try to let your elbows brush against the floor.

➲ Position three

As your hands get even with your face, start to straighten your arms so that they reach out behind your head.

➮ Position four

Stretch out your arms to their full extent. Your shoulders will come up too.

➲ Position five

Take a deep breath, lift your arms, and return to the starting position. Repeat 10 times.

Strengthening the arms

Continue with the arm exercises from level two using weights, and add these. If your arms feel the strain, begin without weights to make sure you are moving correctly, and add the weights as you become stronger.

ARMS – INTERMEDIATE
➲ Position one
Lie on your back with your knees raised and your arms stretched straight up toward the ceiling. Hold a weight in your left hand. Now place your right hand behind your left elbow as a support.

↺ Position two
Breathe in and, as you breathe out, draw your navel to your spine. Slowly lower your left hand (with the weight) toward your left shoulder.

Then bring it back up in a slow movement into the air. Repeat 10 times, and then repeat on the other side.

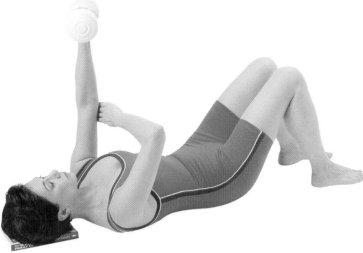

ARMS – ADVANCED
↻ Position one
Lie on your back as in the previous exercise. Stretch your arms up to the ceiling, holding a weight in your left hand only. Place your right hand behind your left elbow as a support.

↺ Position two
Breathe in and, as you breathe out, draw your navel to your spine. Slowly lower your left hand (with the weight) – but this time, across toward your right shoulder.

Bring it back up in a slow movement into the air. Repeat 10 times on each arm.

ARM EXERCISES – STANDING

Here are some more arm exercises, this time in a standing position. It is very important that you start from a secure stance so that you can concentrate on what your arms are doing and not put any strain on your back.

DELTOIDS

The deltoids are the muscles on top of the shoulders and upper arms. Strengthening the deltoids will help to improve your posture, particularly rounded or hunched shoulders, as well as making the joints more mobile.

➲ Position one

Stand about 1 foot (30 cm) away from the wall with your back to it. Place your feet a hips' width apart so that your shoulders, hips, and knees are all in line. Bend your knees slightly and let your entire back lean against the wall.

CHECKLIST

- *Keep your neck, shoulders, and chest open and still throughout.*
- *Go slowly, and with resistance.*
- *Keep your back flat against the wall.*

↻ Position two

Breathe in and, as you breathe out, press down your lats and begin to raise your arms.

Lift both arms straight up to the side, until they are at right angles to your body. Take care not to lift your shoulders. Lower and repeat 10 times.

TRICEPS AND BICEPS

The triceps and biceps are both muscles used in your everyday arm movements. The biceps are at the front and the triceps at the back of the upper arm. This next exercise tones and firms this whole area.

➲ Position one

Stand exactly as you did in the previous exercise, with your shoulders dropped well down and your head and neck free.

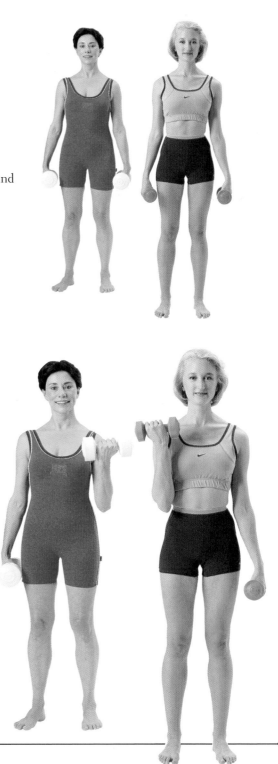

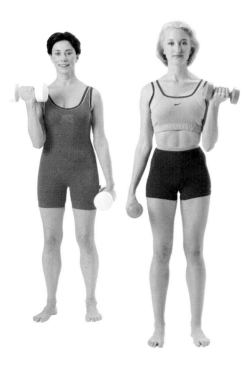

↷ ➲ Positions two and three

Bend one arm at the elbow to raise the weight up toward your chest. As you lower it, start to raise the other arm. Alternate, 10 times on each side.

LUNGE

To exercise your triceps and biceps, stand in the lunge position, so as to prevent the strain of lifting the weight from going into your back. Keep your navel held in throughout, and check that you do not lift your shoulder as you take your arm back.

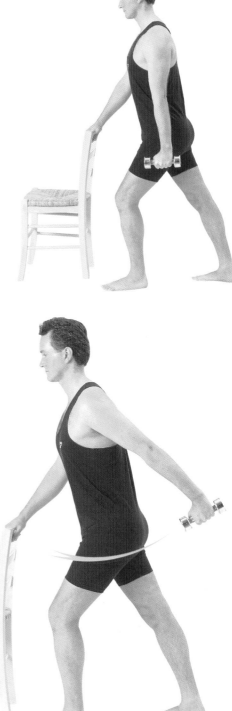

⮎ Position one

Stand away from the wall, with your left hand resting on a heavy piece of furniture. Place your left leg 1 foot (30 cm) in front of the right. Bend your left leg so you are leaning forward in a lunge. Hold a weight in your left hand.

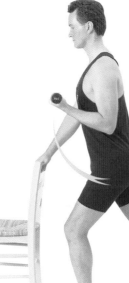

⮌ Position two

Breathe in and, as you breathe out, draw your navel to your spine and pull down your lats. Rotate your left arm so that the palm faces forward, and bend your elbow to raise the weight. Keep your elbow close in to your waist.

⮎ Position three

Take your arm back and repeat 10 times on each side.

Working the legs

REMEDIAL LEGS – ADVANCED

This is the last in this series of remedial leg exercises and this one combines a lift, turning out, and a stretch. Always use one of the earlier remedial leg exercises (see p. 72-73 and p. 98) as a warm-up.

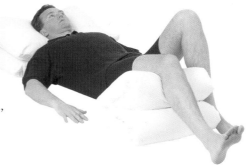

↪ Position one

Lie on your back, with your head and shoulders supported on a large cushion, your right leg over another cushion, and your left leg on the floor.

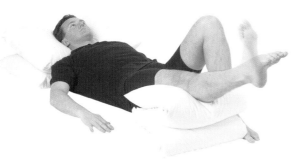

↩ Position two

Breathe in and, as you breathe out, draw your navel to your spine and lift your right leg. When your leg is fully extended, point your foot, then flex it.

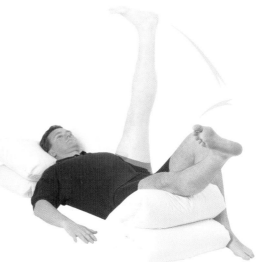

↪ Position three

Turn out your leg from your hip and lift it further across your body toward your left shoulder. This is not a high lift – do not take your leg too far.

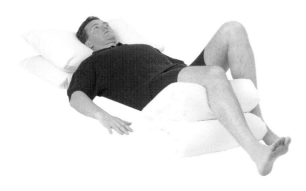

↩ Position four

Take your leg back down to the cushion, turn it in, and lower your foot. Repeat slowly, 10 times on each leg.

Pliés

The plié is, of course, an exercise taken from ballet. It may look like a simple knee bend but it is, in fact, a complex movement when performed properly. Start with just the legs, concentrating on using the leg muscles correctly and keeping the back straight, and add the arm movements later.

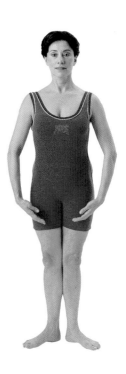

FIRST POSITION PLIÉS

➲ Position one

Stand up straight with your thigh muscles pulled up, and a long spine. Keep your navel held in and squeeze your buttock muscles. Your neck should be long with your head held high. Curve your arms inward. Bring your heels together with the toes pointed out.

↻ Position two

Breathe in and, as you breathe out, bend your knees as much as you can without lifting your heels. As your knees bend, they should remain over your feet. If they roll inward, you are turning your feet out too much; try to narrow the angle. As you bend your knees, turn your thigh muscles out as if you are trying to make the inner thigh face the front. As you bend your knees, your arms lift out to the sides.

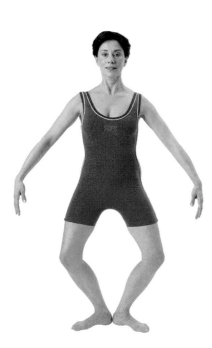

STAY STRAIGHT

- *Never let your heels lift off the floor.*
- *Keep your spine straight at all times – don't arch, lean forward, or round your shoulders. If you do any of these, it may be because you are trying to turn your feet out too much – make the V narrower.*
- *Keep your abdominal muscles held throughout.*
- *Don't let any tension creep into your shoulders.*

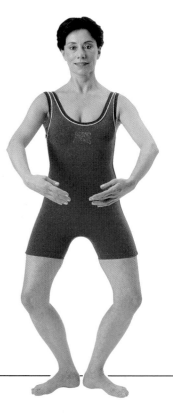

➲ Position three

As you reach the limit of your knee bend, bring your arms forward, still curved, breathe in, and straighten your legs until you are in the starting position. Repeat 10 times.

SECOND POSITION PLIÉS
↻ Position one
Stand with a long back and relaxed shoulders, this time with your feet about 18 inches (30 cm) apart, and your toes pointing out in line with your knees. Keep your navel gently drawn in throughout the exercise and hold your arms in a long curve, with fingers further apart than in the previous exercise.

➲ Position two
Begin to bend your knees, letting your back drop down, again imagining that your inner thigh and buttock muscles are trying to face the front. If your back leans or arches, or your knees roll in, adjust the position of your feet.

↻ Position three
As you bend your knees, start to raise your arms straight out to the sides, with your palms facing forward. As you reach the deepest bend, without lifting your heels off the floor, continue to raise your arms so that they point to the ceiling, but without lifting your shoulders. As you straighten your legs, gently squeezing your thighs together, bring your arms gently back to the starting position. Repeat 10 times.

QUAD STRETCH

For this exercise you will need a strong, fairly high surface (such as a table or kitchen work surface) that will take your weight and allow your leg to reach the floor with a slight bend.

TOO EASY?

If you can do this exercise easily, make it more difficult by placing a rolled-up towel under your leg, just above your knee. If you have difficulty reaching your heel with your hand, use a towel as a loop.

↻ Position one

Lie face down on a table or other surface with your right leg on the table and your left foot on the floor, with a slight bend in your knee. Rest your face on your arms.

↻ Position two

Breathe in and, as you breathe out, tighten your buttock muscles. Slowly raise your heel, bringing it toward your buttocks. Reach back with your hand, take hold of your foot, and gently pull your heel. Hold this position for a few seconds. Breathe in, and lower. Repeat 10 times on each leg.

HAMSTRING STRETCH

Here is a further stretch for the hamstring muscles,
which need to be stretched regularly to counteract the
effects of long-term sitting.

↺ Position one

Sit on a chair with your knees bent at a 90°
angle. Stretch out your left leg and place a
thick book under your heel. Rest both
hands gently on your leg just above your
right knee.

   Take a deep breath in and, breathing out,
stretch your whole spine up, leaning slightly
back and looking up. Keep your spine,
neck, and head in alignment.

↷ ↺ Positions two and three

With your back, neck, and head still in one
piece, breathe out and lean forward, rotating
around the axis of your hip to stretch over your
right leg until you feel the stretch in your
hamstring. Hold the stretch briefly. Breathe in,
and breathe out as you curl your torso forward
over your leg. In a ripple starting from your
pelvis, and running straight up your spine, curl
up until you reach the starting position. Repeat
10 times for each leg.

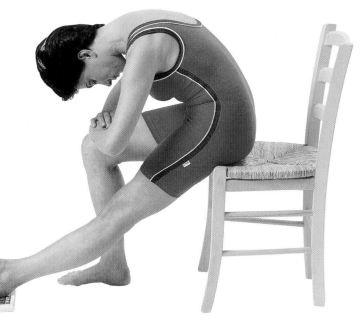

Advanced abdominals

Joseph Pilates' technique teaches you to hold your stomach muscles lightly but firmly as a matter of course, and this advanced oblique and side stretch will test how strong these muscles have become. If this is too much of a strain, you will see them bulge out, putting undue pressure on the stomach muscles and the back. If they do this, stop immediately. Take it slowly and do only one or two repetitions to start. Remember, strain and pain are not the aim.

TAKE CARE!

This is a powerful exercise. Do not hold the position for too long and stop immediately if there is any strain. Check your neck and shoulders for tension as well as your back and abdominals. You can also try this one lying against a wall to help you maintain the correct position.

SIDE STRETCHES
➲ Position one
Lie on your side with your left leg bent and the right one stretched out fully. Hook your right foot under a piece of furniture or ask someone to hold it in place. Your right arm is stretched along your body; the left is bent at the elbow, with your hand resting lightly on your shoulder.

↻ Position two
Breathe in deeply. As you breathe out, feel your upper body lengthen and slowly lift from the floor in one piece. Keep your back straight and your abdominal muscles pulled in. Breathe in and lower. Repeat, building up to 10 times, each side.

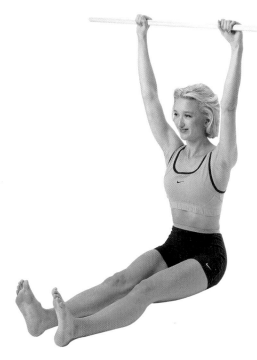

ULTIMATE ABDOMINALS
↺ Position one
Sit on the floor with your legs straight out in front of you, and your feet slightly apart and flexed. Sit up very tall with relaxed shoulders. Hold a pole or a rolled-up towel in your hands, and lift your arms straight above your head without lifting your shoulders.

↷ Position two
Breathe in and, as you breathe out, draw your navel to your spine and start to curl down through your back, gradually lowering your arms.

Continue the curl down until the pole reaches your thighs and the curve extends through your spine and into your neck so that your head drops down slightly.

↪ Position three
Breathe in and, as you breathe out, hold the position of your body but raise the pole as far as you can, if possible bringing your arms back up to your head. Return the pole to your thighs, breathe in, and sit up into position one. Repeat up to 4 times.

Final muscle release

These are the final stages of the cushion squeezes – and hard work! If you are tired by this point, do one of the cushion squeezes from level one or two (see p. 76 or 101).

KNEE SQUEEZE

The effort here should not go into your neck and shoulders; make sure that they stay relaxed throughout this exercise.

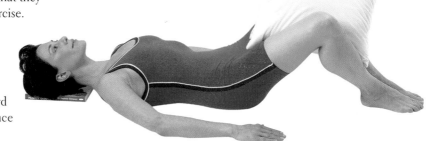

⊃ Position one
Lie flat on your back with your knees raised and a hard cushion between them. Place your hands by your sides.

⊂ Position two
Breathe in and, as you breathe out, draw your navel to your spine and squeeze the cushion between your knees.

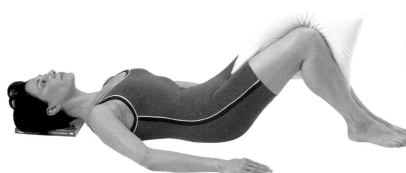

⊃ Position three
As you squeeze, roll your head up, and your shoulders too, if possible, while lifting your arms slightly.
   Breathe in and roll down slowly. Repeat up to 5 times.

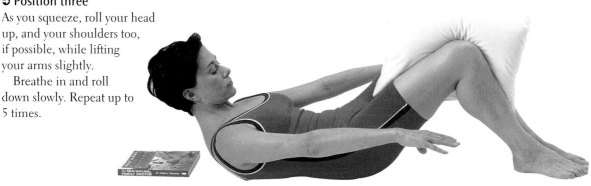

CUSHION SQUEEZE WITH FEET

Again, check that the effort here is made by your legs and abdominal muscles. Don't let it creep into your back, neck, or shoulders.

↻ Position one

Lie flat on your back, with your legs stretched out in front of you. Place your arms by your sides.

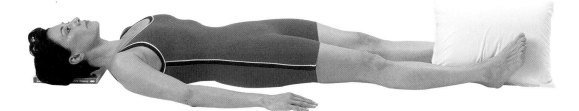

↻ Position two

Breathe in and, as you breathe out, draw your navel to your spine and squeeze the cushion between your feet.

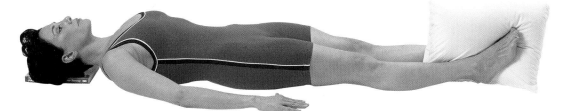

↻ Position three

If you can, try to raise your head up from the floor as you squeeze the cushion. Breathe in to roll down. Repeat up to 5 times.

Appendix

Golden rules of Joseph Pilates' technique

- *Always start with a warm-up.*
- *Take your time! The slower you do these exercises, the better.*
- *Stay in time with your breathing.*
- *Exert all effort when you exhale.*
- *Remember the mantra: Breathe in and, as you breathe out, draw your navel to your spine.*
- *Keep checking your posture.*
- *Stay focused on what your body is doing.*
- *Build up abdominal strength slowly. If your abdominals bulge out during an exercise, stop!*
- *Move your arms and shoulders from your lats and trapezius, not your shoulders themselves.*
- *Follow the instructions for the number of repetitions. Quality, not quantity, is what matters.*
- *Perform the exercises regularly, ideally every other day.*
- *Don't give up – grace and poise can be yours if you persevere.*

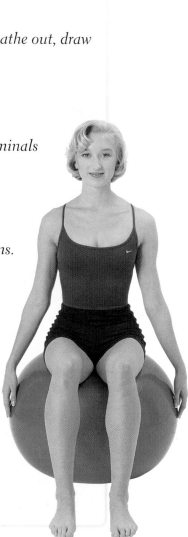

Glossary

MUSCLE GROUPS AND HOW THEY HELP

The **Abdominal** group of muscles extends much further than most people realize, running all the way down to the pubic bone. The main muscle (rectus abdominis) runs all the way down the front of the abdomen and is the one constantly referred to in Joseph Pilates' mantra of "draw the navel to the spine."

➲ The **Oblique Abdominals** help you move from side to side.

➲ The **Rectus Abdominus** bends you forward.

➲ The **Transverse Abdominals** hold in the organs; for example, when you draw your navel to your spine, they hold in the abdominal organs.

➲ The **Bicep Muscles** at the front of the upper arms bend and flex the arms and turn the hands outward.

➲ The **Deltoid Muscles** on top of the shoulders and upper arms move the arms up and down, and extend them out to the sides.

➲ The **Gluteus Maximus** is the main muscle in the buttocks, and is vital for good posture. It is part of Joseph Pilates' girdle of strength, and should be firm. Ideally, it works together with other muscles to create good posture.

➲ The **Hamstrings** run down the backs of the thighs. They bend the knee and support the pelvis. If they are tight, they can put a strain on the lower back.

➲ The **Latissimus Dorsi**, or "lats," are the muscles below the shoulder blades running from the shoulder blades to the pelvis. They support the shoulder blades, and keep them down. Pulling down the "lats" helps to lengthen the spine and initiate good arm movements and posture.

➲ The **Quadriceps**, or "quads," are the muscles along the front of the thighs. They help you bend or extend your leg, lift it forward, flex your thigh, and bend your knees when you walk.

➲ The **Sternum**, also known as the breastbone, joins the ribs together.

➲ The **Trapezius muscle** runs from the shoulders up through the back of the neck. It supports the upper back and arms. It is often very tight, owing to stress accumulated there. In Joseph Pilates' technique, the trapezius and the lats are generally used together to take the strain off the shoulders.

➲ The **Tricep muscles** at the back of the upper arms help the arms to straighten out.

OTHER TERMS

➲ **In one piece**, for example "move your arms backward in one piece," means to move your body in one smooth, graceful movement.

➲ **Draw your navel to your spine** is the phrase you will hear repeated most often in Joseph Pilates' technique. Make sure the effort is when you exhale as you do this. You will feel your pelvis push forward, your gluteus maximus tuck in and tighten, your pelvic floor tighten up (if you are a woman), and the air push out from your lungs. Your posture will automatically improve. If you are not sure that you are doing it correctly, stand sideways at a mirror and practice, noticing the difference in your posture.

➲ **With a long neck** means that, if your shoulders are down, your spine is aligned, your posture is correct, then your neck will be elongated.

➲ **With a neutral spine** refers to the natural curve of the lumbar spine, neither too arched nor too flat.

Useful addresses

PILATES STUDIOS
The Pilates Center
4800 Baseline Road, Suite D206
Boulder, CO 80303
(303) 499-2746
info@thepilatescenter.com

The Pilates Studio
890 Broadway, 6th Floor
New York, NY 10003
(212) 358-7676

The Pilates Studio
2121 Broadway, Suite 201
New York, NY 10023
(212) 875-0189

Ultimate Body Control Studio
30 East 60th Street, Suite 606
New York, NY 10022
(212) 319-6194
info@ultimatebody.com

Momentum
1807 Second Street
Studio 42
Santa Fe, NM 87505
(505) 992-8000
info@momentum-studio.com

Progressive Bodyworks
3620 North East 2nd Avenue
Miami, FL 33137
(305) 438-0555
ana@pro-body.com

PILATES EQUIPMENT
Balanced Body
A Current Concepts Company
7500 14th Avenue, Suite 23
Sacramento, CA 95820
(916) 454-2838
www.balancedbody.com

Acknowledgments

Alan Herdman and Anna Selby would like to thank Karon Bosler, Noelyn George, and Martin Gurnett for modeling; Richard Burns for hair and makeup assistance; Honor Blackman for writing the foreword; Robert Fitzgerald and Carola Trier for being Alan's original teachers; Shirley Hancock for physiotherapy advice; and Balanced Body of California for supplying the equipment featured in the studio section.

Index